FIND THE BLACK BOX

PREVENT NEEDLESS HOSPITAL DEATHS

SECOND EDITION

DR. IRA WILLIAMS

Copyright © 2022 Dr. Ira Williams.

All rights reserved. No part of this book may be reproduced, stored, or transmitted by any means—whether auditory, graphic, mechanical, or electronic—without written permission of both publisher and author, except in the case of brief excerpts used in critical articles and reviews. Unauthorized reproduction of any part of this work is illegal and is punishable by law.

ISBN: 979-8-88640-010-6 (sc)
ISBN: 979-8-88640-011-3 (hc)
ISBN: 979-8-88640-012-0 (e)

Because of the dynamic nature of the Internet, any web addresses or links contained in this book may have changed since publication and may no longer be valid. The views expressed in this work are solely those of the author and do not necessarily reflect the views of the publisher, and the publisher hereby disclaims any responsibility for them.

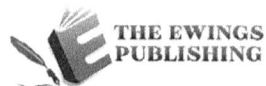

One Galleria Blvd., Suite 1900, Metairie, LA 70001
1-888-421-2397

CONTENTS

Dedication v
Foreword by Robert H. Maguire, Jr vii
Foreword by Ronald Critser ix
2020 Preface xi
Introduction.. xxvii

Chapter 1	Who is Responsible? 1
Chapter 2	What's Missing?...17
Chapter 3	Quality of Healthcare Army of Experts 25
Chapter 4	Quality of Healthcare Improvement Efforts............. 56
Chapter 5	Behind the AMA Curtain.. 100
Chapter 6	What a Collage of Book Reviews Tells Us 129
Chapter 7	Timeline Checklist 165
Chapter 8	The Solution 171
Chapter 9	Conclusion... 187

Notes 195
About the Author 199
Index 2020.. 201

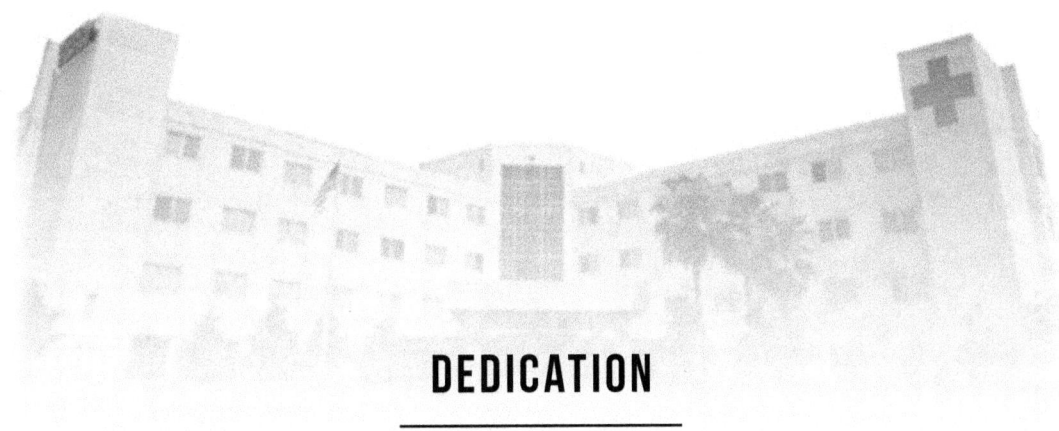

DEDICATION

To those who have died needlessly in our hospitals;

To those who will die needlessly in our hospitals in the foreseeable future;

To those who are left to grieve such tragedy;

To those harmed by medical care, but survive;

To those harmed, and then blacklisted within their medical communities;

To those governors and state legislators who remain clueless regarding healthcare;

To those members of Congress who ignore their responsibility to their states;

To those quality of healthcare experts who deny consideration of all efforts to contribute to making healthcare far better in America

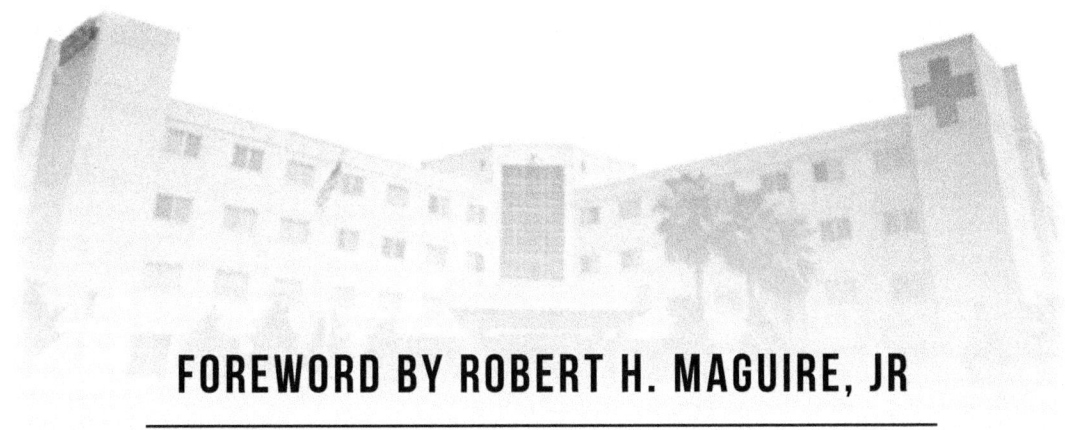

FOREWORD BY ROBERT H. MAGUIRE, JR

If you were to hear in the news—every week—about another commercial airplane crash killing everyone on board, how many weeks would go by before you stopped flying? How long before the general public would stop flying? I predict, not long. Thankfully, the airline industry has a system to prevent such atrocities.

Unfortunately, our healthcare delivery "system" does not have such a system in place. The equivalent of that very same death rate from needless and preventable causes is actually happening within our healthcare delivery "system" right now from coast to coast, in every city and town—and it's getting worse. If hospital deaths were reported the way airline crashes are, there would certainly be public outrage.

In *Find the Black Box: Prevent Needless Hospital Deaths*, Dr. Ira Williams has laid out the necessary steps to replicate the airline industry "system" of transparency and prevention that is totally lacking in healthcare. People in healthcare can provide a litany of reasons to explain why the "healthcare system" is broken, none of which make sense. Their solutions, thus far, don't make sense, either. The system remains "broken" and the deaths keep occurring. Ironically if Dr. William's system were implemented at the state level—as he advocates and knows is the ONLY way—there would be no need for excuses. Every governor, legislator, bureaucrat, citizen, healthcare provider and administrator should read this book.

Status quo is so safe, but not for patients.

For almost a decade, I have worked with Ira Williams as he has helped guide our company and keep us on the right path. I consider it an honor and privilege to also be among his friends. He is truly an asset to the healthcare industry.

Dr. Williams has the vision, integrity, honesty, and determination to offer a solution that would create a healthcare system that works. Rest assured we will be right beside him to help make it happen. Good health is our most important and valuable asset.

~ Robert H. Maguire, Jr., CEO, IntegriSure Healthcare Alliance

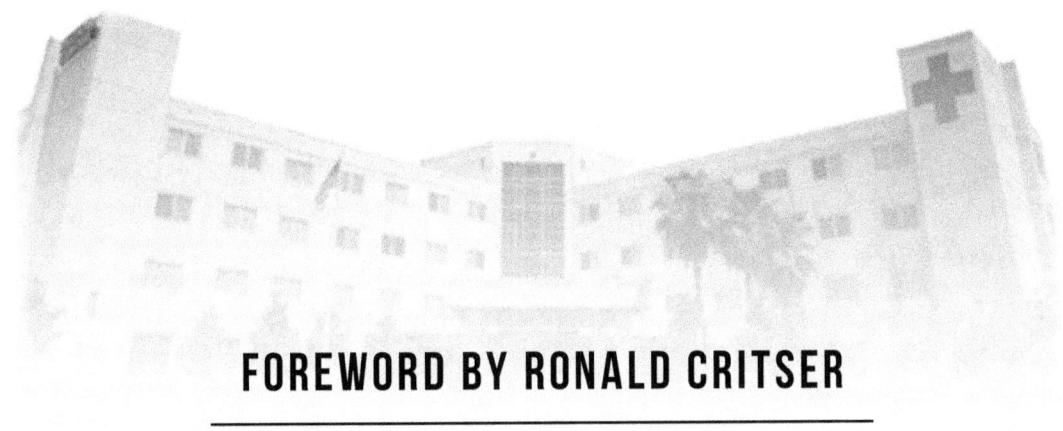

FOREWORD BY RONALD CRITSER

Dr. Ira Williams is a man on a mission.

Having spent thirty years as an officer in the US Marine Corps, I understand what it takes to accomplish any "mission," particularly one wherein human life is at stake. You must first ensure you have adequately defined the goal, dedicated the necessary resources, and done extensive and up-to-the-minute research, paying keen attention to every detail along the way. Such a mission requires arduous training, full commitment, and complete dedication. And those are the skills and vision of my friend, Ira Williams. He was trained in this environment, and he demands of himself that which he would like to see in others.

Perseverance, focus, and the tenacity of a bull dog are some of the adjectives that describe his lifelong efforts to correct the enormous flaws in the American healthcare arena. In this regard, I can only admire him (or maybe pity him), for I don't envy his self-imposed task.

Everything I know and have seen about Ira Williams point to his US Air Force experience as integral to the formation of his farsighted and principled approach to the challenges he has experienced firsthand throughout his medical career. An officer in the military is given great authority commensurate with his/her rank, but in the same breath "held accountable" and "responsible" for the outcome, good or bad. Even when delegating authority to others, the responsibility for all that follows still remains yours. You are accountable! The lives of others depend upon your actions. This theme of accountability is at the heart of Ira's focus in *Find the Black Box: Prevent Needless Hospital Deaths*. He offers an organizational paradigm for the medical community very much like the military's organization—and is further informed by his vast experience and steadfast decency.

I know his passion, and respect all he is attempting in bringing reason and organization into the chaotic world of medicine. I wish him success.

~ Ronald Critser

Colonel Ronald Critser is a pilot and Vietnam veteran. He retired as commanding officer, Marine Corps Air Station, Kaneoha Bay, Hawaii.

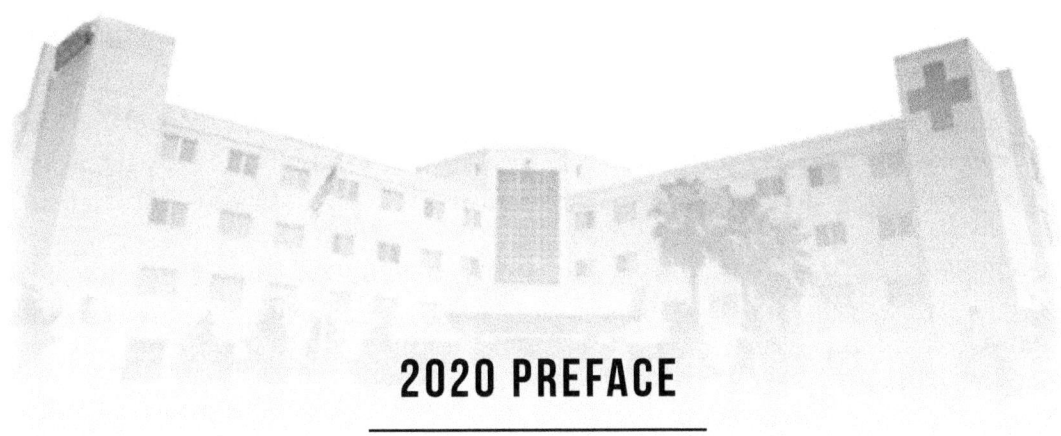

2020 PREFACE

FIND THE BLACK BOX, PREVENT NEEDLESS HOSPITAL DEATHS, and THE SOLUTION NO ONE ELSE IS TALKING ABOUT was first published in 2013, but my efforts to improve the current HEALTHCARE DELIVERY SYSTEM (HCDS) have continued, and my understanding of that enormous, and complex *system* has grown substantially. And the first issue that deserves close consideration is regarding the second sub-title.

THE SOLUTION NO ONE ELSE IS TALKING ABOUT: Not only has no one else been talking about the solution for how to make our current HCDS far better, none of the other Quality of Care and Patient Safety experts who have been publicly promising to create positive change in that *system* have shown the slightest interest in inviting me to join them in their quest for improvement, or even asked for more details about my offering.

Experts (those claiming expertise) not only should be challenged because no one person can know everything there is to know about enormous, complex issues, but every expert should seek to be challenged. Sadly, I have found the entire body of Quality of Care and Patient Safety army of experts to have bear-trap minds, and they are all snapped shut. My books and my offering are meant to be a courteous challenge to other experts, and my intent is to provide positive contributions to their ongoing efforts to make our current HCDS far better, and the next issue I submit for consideration is of the utmost importance.

The Healthcare Delivery System is the Greatest Social Responsibility of every Civilized Nation.

Every civilized nation's HCDS directly impacts every living person from first breathe to last, plus those yet unborn. Yet I believe that every civilized nation's HCDS, particularly within those nations with sizable populations, will be found to be as unorganized, and ineffective where effectiveness is most important as our Nation's current HCDS, and factual evidence to support my contention is clearly evident for those who might seek to recognize such sad facts.

I have been attempting to courteously challenge, and seeking to engage high level political authorities, and healthcare experts since I wrote my 2nd book *MISDIAGNOSED! Why Current Health Care Change is Malpractice* in 2010, and I feel it will be enlightening to share some of my many efforts to help make Your and Your Loved One's HCDS far better.

My Bookends refer to personal efforts in 2010-11, and 2019-20 primarily because of the persons of highest authority I sought to engage with, and share my concerns, and expertise.

2010 Three Events:
"Even if we had a cure for cancer, we couldn't get it to the people because the current system is broken!" Dr. Spence Taylor, Chairman of the Committee seeking to establish a new medical school in Greenville SC in an interview with the Greenville Journal, April.

MISDIAGNOSED! WHY CURRENT HEALTH CARE CHANGE IS MALPRACTICE, my 2nd book was published in September.

Nikki Haley was successfully elected Governor in November, and during her campaigns she said she would listen to anyone seeking to speak with her, and I believed her.

2011: Two Events
"There's no question that our nation's healthcare system is broken." Ingo Angermeier, President/CEO, Spartanburg Regional Hospital, and former President, South Carolina Hospital Association in a article he wrote published in the Greenville Magazine, April.

Governor Nikki Haley provided me with a 10 minute face-to-face meeting in August. I first showed her my back-to-back copies of Dr. Taylor's and Ingo's quotes, and a copy of my latest book, *MISDIAGNOSED!* I then told her that I could provide her with a detailed picture of her State's HCDS. She made no comment, and no offer to meet again.

2013 Governor Haley sent word she could not accept my offer, but no reason was given.

2020: Three Events
CMS Director Verma provided me with contact to her office at a brief face-to-face meeting in Greenville SC in December 2019.

This enabled me to meet with CMS Chief of Medical Staff Dr. Shari Ling, and other staff members at CMS Baltimore Headquarters for 1 hour on March 5, 2020.

I later established contact with CMS Innovation Center Director Brad Smith in May.

My email message to Director Verma, Dr. Ling, and Director Smith in June contained the following: I can provide a process for how to begin to create a 21st century Healthcare Delivery System (doctors, hospitals, and surgery centers). NO response to my offer has been received.

So, during a ten year span my offer to contribute to the efforts to make your and your loved one's HCDS far better have been rejected, first by then SC Governor Nikki Haley, and more recently by CMS Director Verma, and CMS Innovation Center Director Smith, all with NO reason given. But my contact with Nikki Haley had not ended.

STAND for AMERICA, c/o NIKKI HALEY, COLUMBIA, SC.
(requesting donations), and I sent her instead the following letter:

Nikki Haley   July 15, 2020
Concerned Citizen
I doubt you remember our brief meeting in August, 2011 therefore I have included some reminders of that meeting, and my thus far unsuccessful efforts to gain reasonable consideration from decision-makers at Federal, State, and Local levels for the past decade. I have found it exceedingly difficult to find people with open minds.

I know why all of the efforts to improve the quality of care and patient safety have been far more ineffective than promised, and also how to begin to create a 21st century HC Delivery System (doctors & hospitals) worthy of our Nation, but all of the experts appear to be too busy to show interest in my offerings.

Since our brief meeting in August 2011 I have published two new books;
Find The Black Box, Prevent Needless Hospital Deaths 2013 (web site .org)
Healthcare Warriors, Why and How to Become One 2019 (web site .org)

Three Events page is offered as the "bookends" of my efforts to courteously challenge decision-makers in Congress, SC Legislature, Federal Quality of Care Agencies, etc. during the period 2010-2020, and the response has been the same at every level of government; NO interest.

All of the "experts" are forced to agree that the present HCDS is "broken", a very poor word for such a critical understanding, but the word most commonly used. Yet none of those experts have the slightest interest in permitting me to contribute to their efforts to improve the current non-system.

I am writing this with the hope that you will personally have an opportunity to read it, because my plans are to begin to vigorously promote my books and my ideas regarding our current HCDS, why it is broken, and how to begin to correct that critical problem, and given an opportunity I will have this to say about you.

1. I have absolutely no personal animosity toward Governor/Ambassador Haley.
2. I anticipate her 6-year term as SC Governor will be recorded in our State's History books in a very positive manner.

3. In my opinion, Governor Haley *chose to be incompetent* regarding her state's healthcare delivery system, and for more reasons than her failure to give even the slightest consideration to my 2011 offer to her regarding the SC HCDS.

I intend you NO disrespect, but our brief meeting was my first, of many, many attempts to interact with decision-makers at every level of government, and with the same failed result during the past several years.

The Healthcare Delivery System (IMO) is the greatest social responsibility of every civilized nation because that "System" directly impacts every living person, from first breath to last, plus those yet unborn. I can provide a historical timeline, from the first day, of the evolution of our current HCDS, and it is NOT a pretty picture. Our greatest social responsibility has been allowed to evolve with NO master plan, and is now unorganized, and highly dysfunctional, and the reasons why are clearly evident to those who choose to look.

It is evident that you seek to remain a major player on the National scene, and therefore you not only should be challenged, but you should seek to be challenged. And I am taking this opportunity to courteously challenge you regarding our Nation's and our State's HCDS.

I can tell you things about your and your loved one's HCDS that no one else will tell you. But first you must have a desire to gain knowledge of those truths.

My Second Offer: IF you, and others wish to understand why our current HCDS is, and has always been far less than it could or should be, and also how to begin to create a far better system, I am available, but not optimistic.

It must be remembered that there is nothing more difficult to plan, more doubtful of success, not more dangerous to manage then a new system. For the initiator has the enmity of all who would profit by the preservation of the old institution, and merely lukewarm defenders in those who gain by the new one.

Machiavelli

Sadly, his prophetic assessment of human nature is as true today as it was in Florence Italy over 500 years ago, and decision makers still don't get it. No one knows everything about enormous, complex "systems", and that is why it requires a collaboration of efforts to begin to make positive change. I am simply trying to contribute to the efforts to make our Nation's and our State's HCDS far better, and I know how to do that.

Sincerely,
Ira E. Williams

Either her staff in Columbia trashed my letter, or she again felt I deserved NO response.

While my decade-long Bookends demonstrate my attempts to engage persons at the highest state, and highest federal levels of government, and those persons total disinterest, they only represent a very small number of attempts I have made, and continue to make seeking an opportunity to contribute to the efforts to make our current HCDS far better, and since FTBB was first published in 2013 I will limit further examples of my attempts to the past seven years.

2014 I was a Keynote presenter at the 3-day 11th World Healthcare Congress, DC in April, and was probably the only one to speak about each state's responsibility for the HCDS. I also joined the Society to Improve Diagnosis in Medicine (SIDM) and in Sept. attended the 3-day Annual Meeting in Atlanta where I gave a Board member a 2-page paper prior to their morning Board meeting. No Board member spoke to me after they came out of their Board meeting, and I accepted their rejection, and returned home mid-day of the second day.

2016 In July I traveled to DC and attended all day meetings, first at the National Academy of Medicine (NAM), and 2 days later at AHRQ in Rockville MD where I presented both Agencies' Presidents with a 1-page letter offering to provide details regarding my opinion of the 2 Greatest Healthcare Mistakes in the HCDS. My request for consideration was not rejected, but simply ignored by both Federal Agencies' Senior Staff.

2017 I returned to DC for a one-day SIDM meeting at the NAM where I challenged all attendees at the first morning Q&A, and again at the mid-afternoon Q&A. NAM retains videos of their all-day meetings, and my participation should be available if requested.

2018 I challenged my friend and State Representative for his seat in the SC Legislature, not with the thought of winning, but only seeking to participate in an open debate that would allow me to openly discuss the current status of our State's HCDS. But the City Leaders in both Mauldin and Simpsonville (suburbs of Greenville) made sure that there would be no public debate by the candidates. The result was I had wasted a lot of money and good will to no avail. I also released my 4th book *HEALTHCARE WARRIORS, WHY AND HOW TO BECOME ONE* in ebook form only at that time, followed by print in 2019, and audio in 2020.

Governor McMaster, who had succeeded Governor Haley when she became UN Ambassador in 2016 was seeking to remain SC Governor, and he had chosen Pamela Evette, a very successful business woman to be his Lt. Governor. Mrs. Evette kindly allowed me to meet with her and her Administrative Assistant at her business office near Greenville SC in August, before the election. The three of us spent 1 hour in a small room where I presented copies of my 4 books, Dr. Makary's book *UNACCOUNTABLE*, and many documents including the two quotes by Dr. Spence Taylor, and Ingo Angermeier from 2010, and 2011 each stating that the "system is broken", and my offer to then Governor Haley that I could provide a detail picture of the SC HCDS.

The three things that I have taken from that lengthy exchange are; Mrs. (now SC Lt. Governor) Evette said that Dr. Taylor was a friend, I left copies of all of the books, and all of the additional supporting literature, and SC Lt. Governor Evette, and re-elected SC Governor McMaster have never requested that I provide them with additional information.

Dr. Spence Taylor would later become President/CEO of Greenville Health System, the largest such system in the state until his retirement in late 2019, and there is no evidence that Dr. Taylor ever felt he had a responsibility to tell the citizens of South Carolina; How is their HCDS "broken", Why is their HCDS 'broken", and What, if anything, had he and others been doing to "fix" their HCDS? Recognition that our Nation's, and every State's HCDS is, and has always been "broken" for the past several decades is well established. But none of the Quality of Care and Patient Safety experts, including the Federal Quality of Care Agencies seem to want to talk about how to begin to create a far better system that I have been offering for the past decade.

During the past decade I have made many attempts to share my concerns with state legislators, particularly in the Greenville/Spartanburg SC area, and I was always met with complete disinterest. The SC Legislature has 27 standing committees, 14 in the Senate, and 13 in the House of Representatives, and the word HEALTHCARE does not appear on the page. Readers should assume that the SC Legislature is merely a snapshot of other state legislatures, and begin to ask questions where they live. Machiavelli was right, contrarians can expect to receive great opposition, and scant support, as is clearly evident throughout history.

My 2020 BOOKEND

Center for Medicare and Medicaid Services dominates what is allowed, and what is not allowed in most hospitals in the Nation, and their Headquarters outside Baltimore MD is like a giant ant hill with "worker ants" making policy, and shuffling papers from one part of the building to another, but it appears that IF a new idea is not one of their ideas it is not worthy of consideration. CMS Verma became a part of President Trump's Administration because she had been Vice President Pence's Indiana Department of Health Director, and therefore she has great experience regarding the HCDS at the state level, and one should assume that her HCDS had critical shortcomings at that level of patient care. Yet CMS Verma, and her Innovation Center Director Smith have NO interest in what I might have to offer to the efforts to make our current HCDS far better. But I did not end my efforts to courteously challenge "experts" while waiting to see if the CMS decision-makers might open their minds.

MISTREATED, WHY WE THINK WE'RE GETTING GOOD HEALTH CARE – AND WHY WE'RE USUALLY WRONG, Dr. Robert Pearl, M.D. 2017.

This 2020 Preface is being written in November, and I had just belatedly discovered, and read two books, both written in 2017 while writing this Preface.

Dr. Robert Pearl is the former CEO of The Permanente Medical Group (1999-2017), the nation's largest medical group, and former president of The Mid-Atlantic Permanente Medical Group (2009-2017). In these roles he led 10,000 physicians, 38,000 staff and was responsible for the nationally recognized medical care of 5 million Kaiser Permanente members on the west and east coasts.

Named one of *Modern Healthcare's* 50 most influential physician leaders, Pearl is an advocate for the power of integrated, prepaid, technologically advanced and physician-led healthcare delivery. He serves as a clinical professor of plastic surgery at Stanford University School of Medicine and is on the faculty of the Stanford Graduate School of Business, where he teaches courses on strategy and leadership, and lectures on information technology and health care policy. (his web site).

I sent a message to Dr. Pearl on his web site that included the following; I found your book to be an indictment of all of the efforts to improve the quality of care and patient safety during the past several decades, and all of the "experts" who have contributed to those efforts, AND I believe your indictment was proper, and correct. I was surprised, and pleased that he responded.

Hello Dr. Williams,

I'm sorry that what I wrote came across as "an indictment of all the efforts to improve the quality of care and patient safety during the past decades." There are many ways in which we have improved. Having said that, the fact our nation only controls hypertension 55% of the time and screens for colon cancer less than 70% of the time concerns me. And medical errors and avoidable complications from chronic diseases are in the hundreds of thousands. The four pillars I offer have been effective at lowering deaths from heart attacks, sepsis, strokes and cancer by over 30% in various medical groups and organizations.

At the same time, I am always wanting to learn more, so if you have better solutions than the ones I propose, please send them to me and I will read the material in depth.

Thanks
Robbie

Robbie,

Thank you for responding. My intentions are positive. I have written 4 books on the HCDS. All self-published due to a lack of obtaining literary agent support. The consensus is; The System is Broken, but there is little detail discussion about How is it Broken, Why is it Broken, and more importantly, How can we begin to create a far more worthy "System". I can answer all parts of that assessment.

This thing we all have become compelled to call a "system" has always been devoid of any true systematic characteristics, and I can speak to that in great detail, but not in brief soundbites.

Second Great Mistake: States, each state, are responsible to create and maintain an effective HCDS, and no governor or state legislator has ever sought to fulfill that critical responsibility. All medical care is local and states license doctors and hospitals, and surgery centers (we oral surgeons established the credibility of surgery centers long before you "real doctors" recognized their value). Yet during the past ten years I appear to be the only one speaking about the state responsibility.

I was in the CMS Hedqs. outside Baltimore March 5th this year, and I have informed CMS Director Verma, and CMS Innovation Center Director Smith that I can provide a process for how to begin to create a 21st century HCDS, but I have received NO response. I was probably the only speaker at the 11th World HC Congress in DC in 2014 who spoke about each state's responsibility, and I attempted to speak to you, but was unable.

I am just a DDS like your late father (board certified oral & maxillofacial surgeon and anesthesiologist) and I truly believe I have a better understanding of the current HCDS, AND how to begin to create a far better system than anyone else, and every time I say that I mean it as a courteous challenge. NAM has video evidence of me challenging a room full of experts twice at the SIDM meeting on July 17, 2017. Beth McGlynn was there and she accepted a copy of my 3rd book Find The Black Box several years ago. Ask her.

I am attaching My Offer, and hope you will accept. Robbie, I don't mean to offend, and I am not a bomb-thrower. I just want to participate in the efforts to make our HCDS far better, but no one seems to want to accept me.

Ira

Ira

Like you, I don't believe we have a system. In fact, in Mistreated, I label it a 19th century cottage industry. Like you I recognize the issues with trying to provide healthcare to 300 million people and delegating it to 50 different entities (states). [He sees, but doesn't recognize the problem.]

I read a huge amount of material from people with interesting and important ideas -- and learn from all. As I said, I'd be happy to read whatever you choose to send me. My opinions often reflect multiple inputs. I try to credit people in my writing, but find that many ideas overlap.

Robbie

Robbie

Your first few words in your message astound me. Recognition of that FACT by everyone claiming to contribute to the efforts to improve the current non-system must be the first step, but that recognition has only been given passive lip-service since To Err Is Human stated such a possibility on the first page of the Introduction. Dr. Leape told the Senate HELP Subcommittee the plan to adopt safety measures from commercial aviation, and the chemical, and nuclear power industries in Jan. 2000 immediately after publication of To Err Is Human, and twenty years later we are still where we were back then regarding improved quality of care and patient safety at the doctor/patient interface, as you describe in your book.

As a top HC leader in California, can you describe in detail your state's HCDS; identity each component that contributes to that "system", provide some detail regarding each component's contribution, and the Kicker, identify any systematic collaboration between various components necessary to be classified as a true system? We all continue to lie to ourself, and any potential audience every time we use the word system in relation to HC, and wonder why no real progress is being made in the efforts to make the current system (there I go again) better.

And I was disappointed you made no mention of my attachment. Have you had similar offers from others? The next time you reference your desire to help make things better in memory of your father I hope you will re-read my offer list.

Ira

Robbi, I meant to add - I love this, and hope you will continue with the exchange. Ira

Ira

In the book, I point out many of the areas of quality failure and reference "To Err is Human."

I appreciate your offer to provide your thoughts (and data) on the topics. I felt I was responding by leaving it to you to decide what you chose to send me.

I receive dozens of similar offers from smart, insightful doctors and policy experts each week, and wouldn't sleep if I pursued all of the offers similar to yours. I've probably read 50 books written by others and mailed to me since Mistreated. My solution is to leave it to those who write to decide what they feel would be most interesting and helpful.

I think my dad would be pleased with the breadth of feedback I've read, and how I've used it to advance my thinking and writing since the book's publication. Most of those who have sent me material wish I would dive deeper into their recommendations. My approach is what has been labelled "wisdom of the crowd." To that end, I've tried to combine the different ideas with my own. In the end, we don't make much progress in the healthcare system because people (insurers, hospital administrators, specialists, etc.) are not very interested in doing so. As in so many areas, there are multiple solutions that could lead to improvement, but all will fail if people don't choose to pursue them. Like you, at this point in my career (no longer being a CEO) I can encourage and point the way, but I can't force leaders to go forward.

Robbie

Robbie

So I guess you are content with leaving the Public with your book's Sub-Title; Why we think we're getting good healthcare and why we're usually wrong. Tell Beth McGlynn I said hello.

Ira

I hope readers noticed that in his second message to me he stated, "Like you, I don't believe we have a system. In fact, in Mistreated, I label it a 19th century cottage industry." How can experts acknowledge that the current system is a non-system, and continuously ignore the importance of that critical understanding? Use of the word "system" regarding healthcare is a LIE!

EXPERTS with bear-trap minds, and they are ALL CLOSED!

CMS Dir. Verma, CMS Innovation Center Dir. Smith, Dr. Robert Pearl, SC Governor, and former Ambassador Haley, and current SC Governor McMaster, and Lt. Governor Evette show NO interest in the well-documented evidence that your and your loved one's HCDS is, and has always been broken. I have been offering a process for how to begin to create a far better system for the past ten years, and those named above, and many others have shown NO interest.

The second book:

MALPRACTICE, A Neurosurgeon Reveals How Our Health-Care System Puts Patients at Risk, LAWRENCE SCHLACHTER, M.D. 2017

I met Dr. Schlachter, and two other persons for lunch, and discussions regarding my book *FIND THE BLACK BOX* in September 2015, and he stated he was writing a book on medical malpractice at that time. His book, and his experiences as both a surgeon and a plaintiff's attorney in malpractice cases have given him great knowledge and understanding regarding the fundamental unfairness that has been inherent in medical malpractice litigation for centuries in our Nation. But his knowledge and understanding about the current system has not provided him with an understanding of how to replace that system with an effective medical peer review system whereby doctors can fairly judge other doctors regarding questionable patient care. I can provide such a system of fair medica peer review, and said so in my first book *FIRST DO NO HARM, THE CURE FOR MEDICAL MALPRACTICE,* 2004.

I have judged other doctors (MD & DDS) in civil court proceedings regarding questionable patient care, and by doing so, I have come to know how practitioners can fairly judge other doctors. The problem is, that is the last thing doctors would desire to have. Simply stated, doctors are never trained on how to judge other doctor's questionable care because throughout the history of the medical profession doctors' basic inclinations have been to shelter such doctors, and rely on a highly flawed medical malpractice litigation system that allows them to protect their fellow members. In every case in Madison WI that I testified as the second surgeon in malpractice civil court proceeding against MD surgeons involving gross malpractice in each case, the hospital medical staffs, and other doctors, including University of Wisconsin Department heads did everything they could to protect the offending surgeons up to, and including lying under oath. The Medical Profession, including every association, state medical society, and state medical examining board have supported a litigation system that if examined closely might be considered a criminal enterprise. Yet that system has been tolerated by every level of government for centuries.

Another, and possibly the most important book in this Preface: UNDERSTANDING PATIENT SAFETY, Robert M. Wachter, MD, Kiran Gupta, MD, MPH, 3rd Edition, 2018.

This is a large paperback book containing 3 Sections, and 22 Chapters in its 510 pages. Section III: SOLUTIONS contains 10 of those 22 Chapters, and the authors inclusion in the book's PREFACE as to the need for this 3rd Edition is noteworthy.

The first edition of *Understanding Patient Safety* was published in 2007, and the second in 2012. In preparing this third edition five years later, we were impressed by the maturation of the safety field. Between the first and second edition, for example, there were fundamental changes in our understanding of safety targets, with a shift to a focus on harm rather than errors. We saw the emergence of checklists as a key tool in safety. New safety-oriented practices, such as rapid response teams and medication reconciliation, became commonplace. The digitization of medical practice was just beginning to gain steam, but most doctor's offices and hospitals remained paper-bound. Between 2012 and today, the most impressive change has been the wide-spread computerization of the healthcare system.

[Note: there is NO mention of each state's responsibility, and also the consistent use of the word "system" throughout their book while there have been some suggestions that the current "system" is actually a "non-system", a critical realization IF proven to be true, and it is true.]

Dr. Wachter and my brief face-to-face meeting here in Greenville SC in 2010 is described in some detail in this book's 1st Edition INTRODUCTION, and during our brief conversation he admitted he had a problem trying to make his, and other's "solutions" become reality, and I told him, "I can solve that problem". We followed our conversation with a short exchange of email messages, but NO invitation for me to join him in his efforts to make the current system better. Maybe some of my solutions could be included in their next edition.

In 2013 Dr. Wachter gave me permission to use some of his journal articles, and a few of his **AHRQ WebM&M, morbidity and mortality** interviews he periodically conducted with selected patient safety experts during the past decade. Interestingly, at least to me, after I had told him "I can solve that problem" in 2010 he never felt the need to request to interview me. But I hope readers will take particular interest in those few M&M interviews I included.

Semmelweis, Pasteur, Lister, are just a few of the names of those who made great contributions in the on-going efforts to make the delivery of patient care safer, and more effective, and each of those renowned individual's personal histories demonstrate the consistent pattern of obstruction, and denigration evident throughout the history of the medical profession. Contrarian beliefs, even when supported by strong evidence, have consistently been resisted, and opposed, and such unprofessional behavior has continued to be evident during the past decade. But I keep knocking on the door.

I have been saying for the past ten years in my books, personal challenges to Patient Safety experts, and political leaders at every level regarding my belief that there has been NO real, and effective improvement in the efforts to begin to improve the quality of care and patient safety during the past several decades due to the failure by all such experts to recognize, or ignore;

The Two Greatest Mistakes regarding the Healthcare Delivery System:
Each state is responsible to create and maintain an effective Healthcare Delivery System. The current HCDS is, and has always been, devoid of any *systematic characteristics,* and effective accountability will always be impossible to impose without the creation of a clearly defined organizational structure, with effective points of delegated authority necessary for effective accountability to exist.

Dr. Marty Makary's two books, *UNACCOUNTABLE* 2012, and *WHAT PRICE WE PAY* 2019, and Drs. Wachter and Gupta's *UNDERSTANDING PATIENT SAFETEY* 2018, are excellent examples of all of those authors and their books who have been capable of identifying the many problems within the current "system", but have been incapable of identifying the root causes of why NO real improvement in the quality of care and patient safety has been made, and NO suggestion for how to begin to create a 21st century Healthcare Delivery System worthy of our Nation. In fact, they never seem to talk about creating a 21st century HCDS.

Drs. Wachter and Grupta's final statement in their book's CONCLUSION speaks volumes; "We still have much to do before we get there." They recognized "something is still missing" in their on-going efforts to improve the quality of care and patient safety, BUT they still are unable to identify those missing key elements. Perhaps IF Dr. Wachter had taken far more interest in what I might have to offer to their efforts following our verbal exchange here in Greenville SC ten years ago, and invited me to participate in their efforts, we, they, might be further along in their quest for greater understanding.

I am the only quality of care and patient safety expert who has been saying that I can provide clear evidence of what has always been missing in the decades-old efforts to make our current HCDS better, and I am also the only expert who has been saying that I know how to begin to create a 21st century HCDS, but NO ONE seemed interested.

I want to close this 2020 Preface with two final pages in which I seek to identify multiple, specific challenges to members of that vast army of Quality of Care and Patient Safety experts who have been promising quality of care improvements for over three decades, and have little to show for those efforts.

I KNOW WHY OUR CURRENT HCDS HAS ALWAYS FAILED THE PUBLIC, AND I KNOW HOW TO BEGIN TO CREATE A FAR BETTER "SYSTEM". MY PROBEM HAS BEEN MY INABILITY TO FIND EXPERTS WITH OPEN MINDS WHO ARE RECEPTIVE TO BEING CHALLENGED IN A COURTEOUS AND POSITIVE MANNER.

Questions Quality of Care Experts never asked, therefore never answered

1. Is the current HCDS the Greatest Social Responsibility?
2. How is the current HCDS broken?
3. Why is the current HCDS broken?
4. How should a process to improve the current HCDS begin?

Answers
1. The next time a reader or loved one becomes a patient in a hospital they should ask themselves what social responsibility so directly impacts every living person? None.
2. In spite of having the greatest HCDS on the Planet, when individual patient care falls below an acceptable standard of care there is rarely effective accountability. American Medical Association (AMA) has always left the Public with Sue of Forget It, and the AMA definition of medical malpractice is "treatment beneath a standard of care *set by the law.*" The failure to provide effective accountability involving instances of questionable patient care is how the current HCDS has always failed the people it was created to serve.
3. Two Greatest Healthcare Mistakes:
   a. Failure to recognize that since states license doctors and hospitals, each state is responsible to create and maintain an effective HCDS.
   b. Failure to recognize that the current "system" is devoid of any systematic characteristics, and has always lacked a clearly defined organization structure necessary for effective accountability.

4. First there must be recognition of each state's responsibility, and then seek to describe any state's current HCDS by identifying each component that contributes to that system, and seek to identify any evidence of multiple component collaboration that might provide evidence of a true "system". There should be NO attempt to begin to create a new "system" without first creating a well-defined picture of each state's current "system".

"Education is primarily a State and local responsibility in the United States." The Federal Role in Education, U. S. Department of Education, April, 2019.

The same recognition is critically needed regarding our current HCDS.

I can provide the following expertise

Regarding How to Begin to Create a 21st Century HCDS

1. Define and describe the 2 Greatest Healthcare Mistakes regarding the current Healthcare Delivery System.
2. Describe why the multiple Federal Quality of Care and Patient Safety agencies created by Congress have been so ineffective for the past several decades.
3. A detailed picture of any state's current Healthcare Delivery System (doctors & hospitals), including further steps toward creating a new HCDS.
4. A historical timeline of the evolution of our Nation's current Healthcare Delivery System from its first day, and it is NOT a pretty picture.

Regarding How to Provide Effective Medical Staff Accountability

1. A peer review system for how doctors can <u>fairly</u> judge the patient care capability of other doctors, but that is the last thing doctors would wish to have.
2. I can demonstrate unethical and unprofessional conduct within the medical staffs, and by others, in every hospital in the Nation.
3. I can identify the critical medical practitioner responsibility that has been missing or consistently ignored in every hospital medical staff.
4. The imperative responsibilities of every practitioner in every surgery center.
5. How the AMA definition of medical malpractice demonstrates that profession's abandonment of the Public.
6. Clear evidence, in their own words, how the American Hospital Association and their 50 state components have been an enemy of the Public.

Other HC experts have been talking about the Problem(s) – I can, and want to talk about the Solution – but funny thing – I haven't been able to find any other "expert" who wishes to participate in such a dialogue.

I am the author of 4 books on the Healthcare Delivery System, and I challenge other Healthcare experts regarding the above assertions.

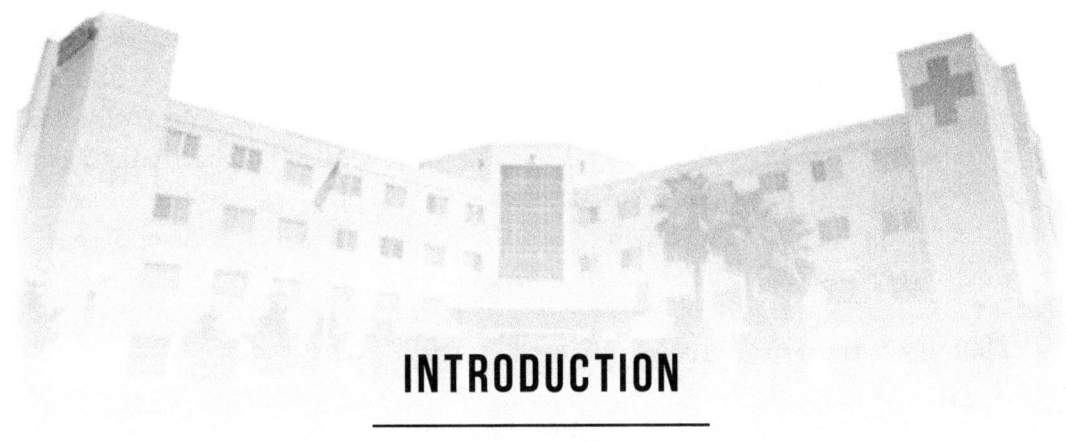

INTRODUCTION

There are 200,000 preventable deaths each year in the US healthcare system, and that is like having 20 Boeing 747 airliners going down each week.

Quality of healthcare experts have recently enlisted both Hero on the Hudson Sully Sullenberger and actor Dennis Quaid in their efforts to preach the need to use commercial aviation safety features in order to improve the quality of healthcare and patient safety since before the beginning of the new millennium But "Sully's" is the first publicly recognized voice from the commercial aviation industry to crossover and actively join in the patient safety efforts. [More on Sully's and Dennis' contributions to patient safety in Chapter 4]

Did you catch the word "preventable" in that tragic analogy? Did that number (200,000 deaths each year) surprise you? . . . the equivalent of ALL THE PEOPLE aboard twenty Boeing 747s dying NEEDLESSLY *every single week*? **Where are the headlines for those daily tragedies that are, and have been, occurring in our nation's hospitals?**

Things are bad in our nation's healthcare delivery system. And what "Sully", Dennis, (and most other Americans) probably doesn't even know fully is just *how bad* things really are *throughout our nation's entire healthcare delivery system.*

This book deals with FACTS, and far too few of those facts have been shared openly with the public. My goal is to provide the facts, in many cases in the very words of those who claim expertise in these matters; and I will connect the dots so that it will be possible to grasp the extent of the problem and understand that a solution is possible—a solution that begins within these pages. There is no time to lose. People are dying needlessly in our nation's hospitals *every single day.*

Fact: Harvard School of Public Health experts in 1990, after four years of research, estimated that the number of needless deaths in our nation's hospitals was estimated to be 98,000 annually and that number more than doubled by early 2012.

That is the wrong kind of progress!

Fact: Experts in 1999 asserted that they had everything needed to provide a 50 percent improvement to that original 1990 Harvard School of Public Health estimate within five years. Yet more than another decade passed; and the rate of needless hospital deaths doubled and continued to rise, rather than fall, despite the efforts of a gigantic army of assorted groups of "quality of healthcare experts" who had been working diligently for decades to reverse that tragic trend.

That too, is the wrong kind of progress!

Fact: Hospitals are the only place in America where an accidental death receives absolutely NO immediate review by any state-level source of authority.

That *fact* should be recognized as unacceptable. Has anyone asked why it isn't? So, who *is* responsible for determining why those thousands of needless deaths continue to occur? And how and when does such review take place? A simple, two-part question will, perhaps, inspire a greater sense of urgency: *Should your loved one become a needless hospital death statistic*, who do you think should review the details and seek the facts regarding that tragedy? And how rapidly should that review occur?

Perspective

In 1990 the number of needless hospital deaths in one year was estimated to be the equivalent to every person listed as killed in combat during three years of war in Korea and ten years of war in Vietnam— combined! By 2012 that tragic annual figure more than doubled; thus the urgent need for questions to be asked and answered. As you will see, the questions are asked and answered within these pages.

Our so-called "quality of healthcare experts" have been questioning their own efforts to reduce the number of needless deaths within our healthcare systems for years. But these experts do not and cannot provide clear, decisive answers as to why their efforts have thus far been so ineffective in reducing the number of sentinel/never events.

A **sentinel event** is defined by The Joint Commission (TJC), formerly the Joint Commission on Accreditation of Healthcare Organizations (JCAHO), as an unanticipated event in a healthcare setting resulting in death or serious injury to a patient, which is not related to the natural course of the patient's illness.

Never event refers to a medical error that should **never** occur, such as a preventable adverse accident or event that results in death or significant disability.

Though our quality of healthcare experts have, thus far, been unable to provide reasons to explain why their efforts have been so impotent, THERE ARE SPECIFIC AND MULTIPLE REASONS. I will outline many of those reasons here and provide a full examination of the "Black Box" pertaining to these events.

The Black Box

After an airplane crash the first item to be searched for and retrieved from the disaster site is the Black Box. This term refers to the equipment in a plane (voice recorder and flight data recorder) that helps crash investigators find out what happened before the crash that led up to, or might have caused, the crash.

With a similar goal in mind—in this case, finding the truth behind the continuing increase in medical errors—*Find the Black Box: Prevent Needless Hospital Deaths* examines and reveals:

- What has always been missing in our nation's healthcare delivery system.
- Why current failed efforts to change that system will continue to fail.
- Why some of those efforts are highly questionable, if not illegal.

And I will do the above using the literature and words of the quality of healthcare experts themselves.

Then what?

Conflict with a positive purpose is the best kind of conflict, and that is my intent with this book. *Find the Black Box: Prevent Needless Hospital Deaths* defines the source of the problem with our current chaotic healthcare delivery system and offers a logical and doable solution that deserves consideration.

This is my third book taking aim at the problems in our healthcare system—problems that continue to cause harm and death every day within our nation's hospitals and surgery centers. My first two books were: *First, Do No Harm: The Cure for Medical Malpractice* (2004), and *Misdiagnosed! Why Current Healthcare Change is Malpractice* (2010).

My passion for this topic is informed by my past military (I am a retired Air Force major and senior navigator/bombardier) and surgery experiences as well as in my career as a physician, a board-certified oral and maxillofacial surgeon, now retired. I consider myself a perpetual student of the US healthcare system, enabling me to challenge, with positive intent, the current ineffective efforts to make our healthcare system better, to identify why those efforts are misdirected, and to offer a viable solution that will save lives.

The Paradox of our Nation's Healthcare System

I will assert and agree that the US has, by far, the greatest healthcare system in the world, regardless of the World Health Organization (WHO) ranking it 37th in a list of 191 countries worldwide. Yet the cost of our healthcare system far exceeds that of any other country, and that cost is constantly increasing and rapidly approaching unsustainable levels. Furthermore, the quality of healthcare within our system has always been problematic, to say the least, as evidenced by the rising number of preventable, NEEDLESS deaths. And there is no evidence suggesting that the quality of patient care will demonstrate significant improvement in the foreseeable future.

So, the product is the best in the world, but far too costly; and the quality of that product has, far too often, been unacceptable. If our nation's healthcare system was a business run by anyone other than politicians who assume there will always be an endless supply of money, it would long ago have declared bankruptcy.

First Major Point for consideration

Each of these two separate, but equally important, aspects of the US healthcare system (cost vs. quality) share a similar characteristic: total chaos. And each *demands* to be considered isolated from the other in order to address their specific form of chaos.

Any form of "cost and access" structure used to pay for healthcare after the fact (whether it is ObamaCare, RomneyCare, ClintonCare, Medicare, Medicaid, whatever—for the insured, uninsured, or uninsurable) must be dealt with completely apart from any consideration of the quality of care within the healthcare delivery system itself.

As someone with expertise in the US healthcare delivery system, I continue to have great interest in these topics. Yet every one of my attempts to discuss the quality of care aspect of healthcare, whether with family, friends, acquaintances, or strangers, turns rapidly to a discussion of "cost and access," or how to pay for healthcare *after the fact*. The healthcare conversation is the same with members of Congress, governors, and within state legislatures. All involved fail to recognize that those two aspects of healthcare are EQUAL IN NEED for dealing with their respective problems, but completely DIFFERENT IN THE TYPES OF EFFORTS REQUIRED TO CONFRONT THOSE NEEDS.

To illustrate: Let's assume a miracle: A perfect solution to pay for healthcare has miraculously been found! Impossible, but permit me to fantasize for a moment.

What then? Sadly, our nation's and every state's healthcare delivery system would still remain as unorganized and dysfunctional as they are today. The reason: the experts trying to improve the current system have been looking in the wrong direction for a workable solution to prevent never events. Discussions about the cost of healthcare serve merely to distract from the issues of safety and medical errors—and the ongoing deaths.

So let's talk about what the quality of healthcare experts have failed to recognize—what has always been missing in our healthcare delivery system.

To talk openly about many of the reasons the quality of healthcare is, statistically speaking, far worse now than it was in 1990, let's go back and briefly review the past track record of those efforts to improve the quality of healthcare and examine why there is no evidence of beneficial improvement.

1. 1990: Healthcare experts estimated that 98,000 preventable hospital deaths occurred annually (the equivalent of 268 patients needlessly dying in our nation's

hospitals each and every day). Note: This research *set a recognized bar* for further attempts to improve the quality of healthcare in America, and was first reported in separate issues of the New England Journal of Medicine as Part I and Part II, February 7, 1991, and Part III, July 25, 1991.

2. 1999: Another group of healthcare experts claimed to have a comprehensive strategy by which government, healthcare providers, industry, and consumers could reduce preventable medical errors–and set as a *minimum* goal achieving a 50 *percent reduction in errors over the next five years*. Note: Institute of Medicine 1999 To Err Is Human: Building a Safer Health System. **never have so few promised so much and delivered so little!**

3. 2012: The needless hospital death rate (the estimate publicly used by Sully Sullenberger and others) reached 200,000 (more than double the original estimate of 98,000 in 1990). No one can question the fact that the very positive progress promised in 1999, and anticipated much sooner, fell far below what our nation should expect from its healthcare delivery system.

Perspective

Earlier, I provided a comparison of the 1990 estimate of needless hospital deaths in one year to the number of people listed as killed in combat during three years of war in Korea and ten years of war in Vietnam—combined! . . . and how that tragic annual figure was estimated to have more than doubled by 2012. I repeat this war analogy intentionally, because, our country was, during that same time period, engaged in two other wars, entailing the tragic loss of hundreds of lives each year. But even those figures pale when compared to the carnage that occurred on a daily basis within our nation's hospitals—and continued UNABATED for more than two decades. **Where is the outrage?**

People enter hospitals in America with the expectation that they will be safe. They end up as patients in our hospitals because they are sick or injured—not as casualties of a war abroad. But our hospitals are not safe, and never have been, and the increasing numbers of needless deaths are the evidence.

What will it take for the American public and their leaders to recognize a crisis?

The 1990 statistic mobilized a great effort to make things better; but many years passed, and things became far worse. And there is more, much more, that continues to fly under the "healthcare radar" with a deafening silence.

On May 20, 2009, almost two decades after the original 1990 research, a co-leader of that research, Lucian Leape, along with Janet Corrigan, a co-editor of the 1999 publication, *To Err Is Human,* gave a presentation in Washington DC entitled, "Reflections on the Past 10 Years: Why Have We Not Gotten Further?" Unfortunately, their joint presentation was only offered to an exclusively select group. Also unfortunate, their "reasons" for the monumental failure to even come close to their promised five-year goal in improving the quality of healthcare was NEVER MADE PUBLIC.

I would find it interesting to compare their "reasons" for lack of success in their efforts and my own reasons for the same failures. I suspect that our reasons would differ dramatically. I will share my reasons here, not the least of which is that this type of information should not remain a secret from the people who rely on our healthcare system in matters of life and death every single day!

Connecting the dots

The previous summary of key events is a sanitized version of the attempts by a multitude of quality of healthcare experts since 1990 to make our nation's healthcare system safer and more effective. The fact that there have been so many more needless hospital deaths each year than there were more than twenty years ago should lead to an obvious question: Are the quality of healthcare experts' efforts misdirected?

While the quality of healthcare experts have given no public evidence of any questioning of the thrust of their efforts until very recently, this book is predicated on the belief that the absence of positive improvement in the quality of healthcare is a direct result of their failure to recognize the responsibility of every single state in the creation of an effective healthcare delivery system. So I will go back and start again at the beginning of this review of two decades of questionable effort.

Physicians Troven Brennan and Lucian Leape, were co-leaders in that four-year study of hospitals in Upstate New York that began in 1986. Their results were first reported in 1990, and later published in separate issues of the *New England Journal of Medicine*. That study set the statistical bar at an estimated annual rate of 98,000 needless hospital deaths.

The following several paragraphs are quoted from the National Academies Press web site describing the "Quality of Healthcare in America" project in 1998 initiated by the Institute of Medicine and reported in To Err Is Human in 1999.

> Experts estimate that as many as 98,000 people die in any given year from medical errors that occur in hospitals. That's more than die from motor vehicle accidents, breast cancer, or AIDS—three causes that receive far more public attention. Indeed, more people die annually from medication errors than from workplace injuries. Add the financial cost to the human tragedy, and medical error easily rises to the top ranks of urgent, widespread public problems.
>
> *To Err Is Human* breaks the silence that has surrounded medical errors and their consequence—but not by pointing fingers at caring healthcare professionals who make honest mistakes. After all, to err is human. Instead, this book sets forth a national agenda—with state and local implications—for reducing medical errors and improving patient safety through the design of a safer health system.
>
> This volume reveals the often startling statistics of medical error and the disparity between the incidence of error and public perception of it, given many

patients' expectations that the medical profession always performs perfectly. A careful examination is made of how the surrounding forces of legislation, regulation, and market activity influence the quality of care provided by healthcare organizations and then looks at their handling of medical mistakes.

Using a detailed case study, the book reviews the current understanding of why these mistakes happen. A key theme is that legitimate liability concerns discourage reporting of errors—which begs the question, "How can we learn from our mistakes?"

Balancing regulatory versus market-based initiatives and public versus private efforts, the Institute of Medicine presents wide-ranging recommendations for improving patient safety, in the areas of leadership, improved data collection and analysis, and development of effective systems at the level of direct patient care.

To Err Is Human asserts that the problem is not bad people in healthcare—it is that good people are working in bad systems that need to be made safer. Comprehensive and straightforward, this book offers a clear prescription for raising the level of patient safety in American healthcare. It also explains how patients themselves can influence the quality of care that they receive once they check into the hospital. This book will be vitally important to federal, state, and local health policy makers and regulators, health professional licensing officials, hospital administrators, medical educators and students, health caregivers, health journalists, patient advocates—as well as patients themselves.

Two key points must be recognized from *To Err Is Human*:

1. The estimate of 98,000 needless hospital deaths referred to in *To Err Is Human* was taken from the Brennan, Leape, et al., study first reported in 1990.
2. The book asserts that "Given current knowledge about the magnitude of the problem, the committee believes it would be IRRESPONSIBLE TO EXPECT ANYTHING LESS than a 50 PERCENT REDUCTION IN ERRORS OVER FIVE YEARS.
   [emphasis mine]

   Fast forward to the National Patient Safety Foundation Pre- Conference meeting in Washington DC on May 20, 2009, wherein the title of the first session (presented by Lucian Leape and Janet Corrigan) was called "Reflections on the Past Ten Years: Why Have We Not Gotten Further?"

Then Sully comes along in 2012 and says that the number of people *needlessly dying* in our nation's hospitals is equal to twenty Boeing 747 airliners going down each week.

I keep asking, what are their reasons for, "Why Have We Not Gotten Further"?

Others Weighed In

A two-year Rand Corporation report in 2004, "The Quality of Health Care Delivered to Adults in the United States," was the first comprehensive study of healthcare provided in metropolitan areas. The study noted that Americans get substandard care for their ailments about half the time, even if they live near a major teaching hospital. The inadequate treatment leads to "thousands of needless tests each year," according to the lead author, Dr. Elizabeth McGlynn, a researcher at the RAND Corporation. "Only a fundamental redesign of the health system will improve the situation." She noted that this is asking for "a tremendous cultural shift." (In 2011 Dr. McGlynn was named director of The Center for Effectiveness and Safety Research at Kaiser Permanente.)

What improvement might a similar study reveal today?

National Quality Forum (NQF) reported in 2008 that "A 1999 Institute of Medicine report estimated that as many as 44,000 to 98,000 people die in US hospitals each year as a result of medical errors – more than deaths caused by car accidents, breast cancer, or AIDS. In the intervening nine years, that statistic has not improved as much as one would hope. Patient safety measures indicate that our nation is *improving in this area only 1 percent each year.* [emphasis mine]

So, in 1999, "they" promised a 50 percent improvement in five years; and in 2008 "they" estimated achieving "only 1 percent improvement per year." I don't know how anyone can measure a single percent rate of change, in either direction in our nation's healthcare delivery system, but apparently "they" can. At that rate, our great grandchildren might be finally gifted with that promised 50 percent improvement in patient safety in our hospitals.

Since *To Err Is Human*, the quality of healthcare experts have actively been coalescing their efforts through "harmonization" (their word). They speak of harmonizing their message(s) since so many groups are saying the same thing while using different words.

Confirmation bias has become the mantra of the quality of healthcare experts, and that mantra has unfortunately replaced the time-honored tradition of scientific advancement being achieved by positive-intended challenge. The medical profession's "code of silence" has permeated the quality of healthcare experts, and to the detriment of all they seek to serve.

Quality of healthcare experts have, in essence, become a cottage industry that in too many ways has become more obsessed with their being recognized as the source of all quality of healthcare understanding than in the effort to make our nation's healthcare delivery system far safer. Conflicting contributions and contrarian viewpoints are seemingly never sought or tolerated.

With positive intent, I seek to challenge the quality of healthcare experts based upon their failure to recognize the state responsibility in regard to the healthcare delivery system and their well-documented record of "Why Have We Not Gotten Further?"

The central point of this complex issue is not only that our personal healthcare delivery system is sure to reach out and grab each of us at some time in our future, but that same system will also directly impact the lives of our children and grandchildren. This subject is far too serious to every American to be continually and passively ignored by our nation's decision makers, yet the overwhelming roar for healthcare change is focused almost solely on how to pay for healthcare after the fact.

For example, people in the Greenville, South Carolina area (my hometown) were given a strong dose of the quality of healthcare reality in our community by a highly qualified source as quoted in the weekly *Greenville Journal* in April 2010: "Even if you cured cancer you couldn't get it to the people because the medical system is broken." That expert was Dr. Spence Taylor, chairman of General Surgery, Greenville Hospital System, and operations director of the new USC School of Medicine/Greenville Development Team. The editor/journalist recording his thought-provoking statement apparently didn't even blink an eye at Dr. Taylor's astounding acknowledgment, but proceeded to skip a line and begin a new segment in her otherwise glowing article on the Greenville area's new medical school.

"The medical system is broken!" should not so easily be rolled off of someone's tongue and be passively ignored, particularly when it's from such an esteemed source as Dr. Taylor. Yet it has been completely ignored by every decision maker and community watchdog in both the Greenville area and the state capital.

Some who read this book will have already experienced the tragedy of a needless hospital death in their family. Other readers may face such a fate in the future. The numbers have been "out there" for more than two decades, but the numbers are only numbers until someone puts a name and a face on each of them, which should lead any thinking person to;

That fact still remains: hospitals are the only place in America where an accidental death receives no immediate, detailed review by a source of state authority! That fact is a disgrace, but it is also a look behind the curtain of our current unorganized and dysfunctional healthcare delivery system.

Our nation's healthcare delivery system is becoming more dysfunctional each year, and there are clearly evident reasons why. But no one is talking about the specific fundamental flaws resulting in that ever-increasing dysfunction.

As I boldly stated at the start, I know why our needless hospital death rate is greater than it was over twenty years ago, and also why there is little potential for reversing that deadly trend while relying on more of the same, or similar efforts of the past twenty-plus years. Evidence for my assured lack of optimism for beneficial improvement in the quality of healthcare is contained in a portion of the above quote from *To Err Is Human*: ". . . the committee lays out a comprehensive strategy by which government, healthcare providers, industry, and consumers can reduce preventable medical errors."

Anyone who believes a consortium of government (federal, state, or a combination), healthcare providers, industry, and consumers can conjure up a magical way to vastly improve the quality of patient care in our current healthcare system should be careful what they pray for, while ignoring the simplistic nonsense contained in that statement.

I want to share a brief, but most informative, one-on-one conversation I had here in Greenville, South Carolina, with Robert M. Wachter MD, professor of Medicine and chief of the Division of Hospital Medicine at the University of California—San Francisco, and the person who coined the term "hospitalist" (more on this later). Dr. Wachter's presentation at Greenville Hospital System on September 30, 2010, was open to the public, and he was introduced as "one of the premier experts in the world regarding patient safety."

Dr. Wachter's presentation was entitled, "What We Need to Know and Do to Cure Our Epidemic of Medical Mistakes." I was the first person to capture his attention as he concluded his remarks and descended from the stage. We stood shoulder to shoulder close to the side of the steps to the stage and had the following cordial exchange (I also gave him a copy of *Misdiagnosed!*):

IW: "Dr. Wachter, you speak of systems errors, and in my two books I speak of individual practitioner errors. If we brought the two together we would really have something." Then I asked, "How do you get your system of systems errors to all of the hospitals in the nation?"

Dr. Wachter: "That's a problem." IW: "I can solve that problem." Dr. Wachter: [Silence]

Because others were waiting to speak with Dr. Wachter, I stepped aside and quietly left the room; but that brief exchange I just shared with "one of the premier experts in the world regarding patient safety" stayed with me.

Early the next week, I emailed Dr. Wachter: "Did you read my book I gave you, *Misdiagnosed!*; and if so, what do you think?" I also added, "I am as passionate as anyone you know in wanting to contribute to making healthcare better. Is there room for me under your big tent?"

Dr. Wachter emailed a reply several hours later: "Yes, I read your book. You make some interesting suggestions." He added, "I don't know of anything now, but I will keep you in mind."

Three years later and I have yet to hear from Dr. Wachter, except for the permissions he granted for later in this book, or to be invited to visit his big quality of healthcare tent.

My question, "How do you get your system of systems errors to all of the hospitals in the nation?" and Dr. Wachter's response, "that's a problem" goes to the very heart of "Why Have We Not Gotten Further?" There is no mechanism for relaying change to every healthcare system in the country.

Interestingly, Dr. Wachter made no reference to such a problem in his presentation, "What We Need to Know and Do to Cure Our Epidemic of Medical Mistakes" that day in Greenville, South Carolina.

The current vast army of quality of healthcare experts cannot tell the public how they can get their offerings for beneficial patient safety change into every hospital in the nation—because they don't know themselves! And their efforts, to date, prove their lack of understanding.

Various sources estimate the number of hospitals nationally to be somewhere between 5,500 and 6,000. Other sources estimate the number of surgery centers to be rapidly approaching the number of hospitals. People needlessly die in both types of patient care facilities, but our quality of healthcare experts completely ignore a major portion of our current healthcare system: surgery centers. None of them talk about the surgery centers, none except me, a board-certified oral and maxillofacial surgeon. Oral surgeons pioneered the benefits of surgery centers prior to World War II.

There are fundamental flaws inherent in every aspect of our current healthcare delivery system (which is actually a non-system, but more on that later) and those fundamental flaws continue to be either passively ignored or unrecognized.

A nationally-recognized patient safety activist, after reading my second book, *Misdiagnosed: Why Current Healthcare Change is Malpractice*, told me, "Ira, your problem is that you are trying to tell everyone else they are wrong."

That person's well-intended critique was only half right. I am just the messenger. The facts, as demonstrated throughout this book, collectively illustrate how the current quality of healthcare army of experts have completely failed to recognize that all of their efforts for the past two decades have been like trying to play bridge without all the face cards.

Ignaz Semmelweis was a nineteenth century obstetrician whose name has surprisingly been identified by several of the quality of healthcare experts in recent years as the doctor who introduced hand-washing to medical care, and like that patient safety activist's critique of me, their description of Semmelweis is also only half right. I say it's surprising that his name has been used because the medical leaders of his day, both in Vienna and later in Budapest, rejected Semmelweis and his patient safety efforts. He ended his life in an insane asylum. More on Semmelweis later, because he and his complete story are so very important. Surgeon Joseph Lister, who always gave credit to Semmelweis, was able to finally introduce that life-saving practice of both hand and instrument washing (still highly relevant) first in England, and far away from those medical leaders in Vienna and Budapest.

The Point

The current estimated annual rate of needless hospital deaths is far greater now than was estimated, and accepted as the baseline over two decades ago. The enormous size of the current army of quality of healthcare experts, and the volumes of literature presented as solid methods for creating quality improvement and greater patient safety beginning with *To Err Is Human,* stands exposed by the undeniable fact of that first statement. There is no hard evidence of measurable improvement in either the quality of healthcare or in greater patient safety. At some point, someone must ask hard questions and demand complete, detailed answers.

The medical leaders in Vienna and Budapest had bear-trap minds that were snapped shut. Those leaders preferred to continue to do things their old way, regardless of the number of lives they would continue to lose, rather than consider a different, and by then, proven method of patient care.

I know why the current efforts of that army of quality of healthcare experts have been proven to be inadequate for their task. I have reached out and made direct contact with most of the quality of healthcare expert leaders who will be named in this book, and none of them have been receptive. Sadly, it is difficult, if not impossible, to find open minds within the leadership of the quality of healthcare army of experts.

Unfortunately, I anticipate that the quality of healthcare army of experts, i.e. Dr. Wachter, etc., will continue to exclude my effort to contribute to improving healthcare in America. What the quality of healthcare experts fail to understand is that my attempt to help create an organizational structure for our healthcare delivery system is exactly what they have always needed in order to allow their improvements to take effect in every hospital and surgery center in America. Dr. Wachter demonstrated that lack of understanding with his answer to me, "That's a problem."

But there is far more to the intent of this book than my passionate and fundamental differences with the past efforts of the quality of healthcare experts in their misguided attempts to incrementally change an unorganized and dysfunctional non-system. William Anthony Hay, in his *Wall Street Journal* Bookshelf review of J.H. Elliott's book *History in the Making* on January 4, 2013, expressed my multiple intents in this book much better than I ever could.

The complexity of writing history is a recurring theme in Mr. Elliott's memoir. He writes that, 'no narrative is ever fully comprehensive, no explanation total, and the balance between description and analysis is painfully elusive.' The best historians can do, he suggests, 'is to sift through the sources and provide a plausible reconstruction of the past, one that is so effectively presented as to draw the reader in and make a persuasive case for particular version of events." That is precisely what I am attempting to do within these pages.

Therefore, I describe the multiple intents of this book as:

- A plausible reconstruction of the past history of healthcare in America and efforts to improve the quality of care.
- A critique of the quality of healthcare experts' efforts to improve that system, providing you with many of the sources' documents in their own words, and showing how the evidence of their results, thus far, cries out for close examination.
- An offer of a far better solution to the problem.

When I told Dr. Wachter, "I can solve that problem," I meant it!

When he said NOTHING, and then later said, "I will keep you in mind," only he can say what he meant. The American public has a right to be in on the conversation. Within Dr. Wachter's circle of experts, there is often an acknowledgment of the need for an open debate, but rarely, if ever, does such a debate take place, as debates should, between qualified sources with widely divergent viewpoints.

This book offers a courteous challenge for such a debate. I respectfully offer myself as qualified to assume the contrarian position.

If you want to know why our healthcare delivery system is so very sick and also why that system has always been sick, but keeps getting sicker, keep reading. But please keep both Mr. Elliott's and Mr. Hay's insightful comments in mind. Writing a book about the problems in our current healthcare delivery system is like assuming one sees all they need to know about an iceberg by what they see above the surface of the water. This book paints a picture of our current healthcare delivery system, and its plethora of problems; but sadly that picture is not very pretty.

Too many highly educated, highly dedicated people are sincerely trying to change and improve a huge, complex system none of them can describe—in detail. And they wonder why their collective efforts of the past two decades demonstrate only slight clusters of improvement and NO fundamental change.

Hubris (excessive pride or self-confidence) must be one of the strong characteristics of anyone who seeks to "change" a huge, complex system those innovators can't first describe. Unfortunately, that is an accurate description of the quality of healthcare army of experts and their efforts during the past two decades.

> "It must be remembered that there is nothing more difficult to plan, more doubtful of success, nor more dangerous to manage than a new system. For the initiator has the enmity of all who would profit by the preservation of the old institution and merely lukewarm defenders in those who gain by the new one."
>
> ~Niccolo Machiavelli.

I do not seek to "*re*-organize" our current healthcare delivery system, because we have never had a truly organized healthcare delivery system in the first place. There is nothing systematic about our current system. I seek to contribute, with others, in an effort to finally, for the first time in our nation's history, begin to CREATE a healthcare delivery system worthy of our great nation so that new system might function in a far more effective and efficient manner for all.

I invite you to join me in such an effort. Some hints as to what, up to now, have received little, if any, public exposure or recognition:

- Major components of the army of quality of healthcare experts, in their own words (key portions of source documents are conveniently included within this book so that readers can immediately access the information).
- Comparison between what they say, and have been saying for so long, with what others have offered.
- Sully Sullenberger and three cohorts' efforts to create a new, federal, patient safety bureaucracy that is theoretically interesting but in reality nonsense.
- How the AMA, all fifty state medical societies, and some state medical examining boards (as needed) have united to *corrupt* (the right word) the medical malpractice litigation system.

- How brief reviews of several books taken together provide an enlightened perspective on the quality of healthcare in America.
- A timeline checklist of the efforts to improve the quality of healthcare and patient safety since the mid-1980s.
- Finally, a solution, far different than previously offered or imagined, that can provide what has always been missing in the non-system we have called our nation's healthcare delivery system.

Find the Black Box

Dr. Lucian Leape, co-leader of the four-year research project that provided the 1990 estimate of 98,000 needless hospital deaths annually, is credited with originating the concept that quality of healthcare experts should (must) mirror the safety measures of commercial aviation. *If* the full benefits of pilot competence in the airline industry were incorporated into the practice of medicine, as they should be, the quality of patient care would be dramatically improved.

One of the most productive safety measures of that industry has been the black box equipment contained in all commercial aircraft in recent decades. One of the greatest deficiencies in our nation's healthcare delivery system has been the absence of similar "black boxes" when disaster strikes in that "industry."

Find the Black Box: Prevent Needless Hospital Deaths goes to the very heart of the needless and preventable hospital deaths that are rampant throughout the US healthcare delivery system. As in many airplane crashes, finding the healthcare black box is easier said than done, but more on that in Chapter 1.

> "You can avoid reality, but you cannot avoid the consequences of avoiding reality."
>
> ~ Ayn Rand

My instincts as an Air Force bombardier compel me to focus on as precise a target as possible; and, regarding the healthcare delivery system, that target is as clear and precise as: two plus two equals four. *Find the Black Box* will demonstrate not only how there is nothing systematic about our current healthcare system, but also how quality of healthcare experts and decision makers at every level continue to avoid the reality that the healthcare delivery system is a STATE responsibility.

"Sully's" dramatic and sadly accurate assessment of the quality of healthcare in America speaks to the enormous degree of the "problems in healthcare" and illustrates how profoundly unproductive the efforts to improve the quality of healthcare have been, and continue to be. **Find the Black Box** reviews many of those unproductive efforts, describes the fundamentals that have always been missing *and unrecognized* in those efforts, and then offers a logical and doable, multi-step process to FINALLY begin to create a healthcare delivery system worthy of our nation.

Imperative: Keep your eyes on the FACTS, and not on the messenger; and constantly remember the focus of this book is on yours and mine, your children's, and your grandchildren's healthcare delivery system—the system that each of us enters when sick or injured, and the system that someday will likely "welcome" us all. But unfortunately, entering that system is like playing Russian roulette with more than one bullet in the six chambers.

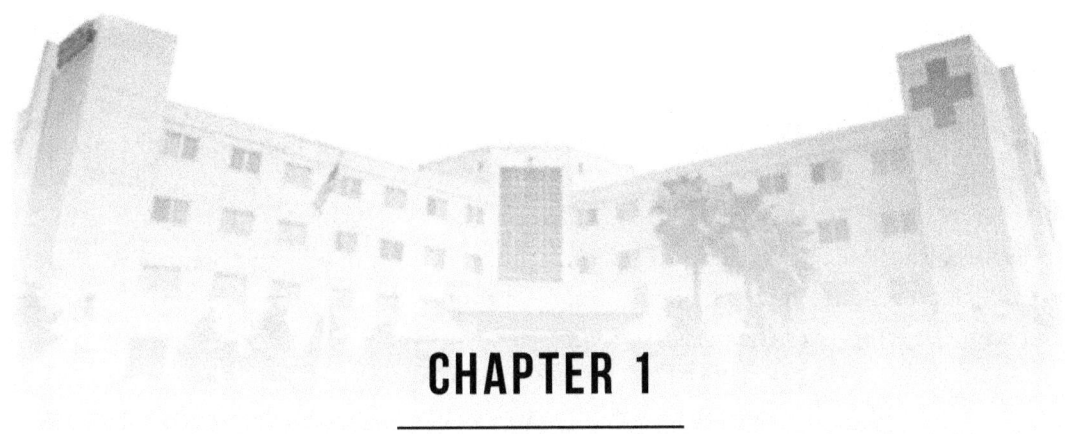

CHAPTER 1

WHO IS RESPONSIBLE?

STATES are responsible for our nation's healthcare delivery system. It's that simple. Why? Because of two *fundamental facts*:

(1) States license doctors, and (2) all medical care is local.

I assume no one will attempt to deny that states license doctors, therefore I will focus on the second point for a moment with a quote from a *New York Times* OP-ED article, "10 Steps to Better Healthcare" by Atul Gawande, Donald Berwick, Elliott Fisher and Mark McClellan, all medical experts, in August 2009.

"But all medicine is local. And until a community confronts what goes on in its own population – to the point of actually seeking the data and engaging those who can solve the problem – nothing will change.

YES, I say!!! From the horses' mouths! I assume no one will wish to dispute those words from these impeccable medical sources.

However, I see two problems with any community trying to find what is needed to confront such matters.

First, these four experts fail to explain exactly how any community can CONFRONT, OBTAIN DATA, and ENGAGE THOSE WHO CAN SOLVE THE PROBLEM.

Second, since MORE PEOPLE ARE DYING NEEDLESSLY in our nation's hospitals now than were dying needlessly over two decades ago, where and how might community members engage those who can SOLVE the problem?

More importantly, can those four medical experts identify such a healthcare "problem solver" in any community in the nation? They couldn't then, and they still can't today.

There are too many "quality of healthcare experts" out there who are speaking out of both sides of their mouths—but that is just my opinion.

Chronological Review of Key Facts

1990: Healthcare experts estimated that 98,000 preventable hospital deaths occurred annually.

1999: Healthcare experts (in *To Err is Human*) claimed to have a comprehensive strategy to reduce preventable medical errors, and set a minimum goal of achieving a 50 percent reduction in errors over the next five years.

2008: National Quality Forum (NQF) reported that patient safety measures in our nation are improving only 1 percent each year.

2009: National Patient Safety Foundation presentation "Reflection on the Past 10 Years: Why Have We Not Gotten Further?" by Lucian L. Leape, MD (co-leader of the 1990 report) and Janet Corrigan, PhD, MBA (co- editor of *To Err Is Human*) is made to a select, non-public audience.

2009: Doctors Gawande, Berwick, Fisher, and McClellan assert that ALL medical care is local.

2010: Dr. Spence Taylor, Greenville Hospital System, says, "Even if you cured cancer, you couldn't get it to the people because the medical system is broken."

2012: Sully Sullenberger says, "There are 200,000 preventable deaths each year in the US healthcare system. It is like having 20 Boeing 747 airliners going down each week."

"Our" Problem

No one, and I do mean *no one*, within the entire army of quality of healthcare experts ever provided the slightest evidence of any recognition (since all medical care is local and state's license doctors) that each of the fifty states bears the major responsibility for the creation and maintenance of an effective healthcare delivery system. Thousands of patients continue to die needlessly in our nation's hospitals (and surgery centers), and no one appears to recognize those two *fundamental truths* about healthcare.

Back in 2010, when I asked one of the "premier" patient safety experts in the world, Dr. Robert M. Wachter, "How do you get your system of systems errors to all of the hospitals in the nation?," he acknowledged, "That's a problem."

Now my (our) "problem" is this: How do we get the army of quality of healthcare experts, and everyone else, to recognize that the healthcare delivery system is a state responsibility—so that states can actually then accept that responsibility? I have three reasonably simple steps to offer those who wish to better understand the state responsibility.

Finding the Black Box

The tragic loss of the Air France airplane that crashed in the South Atlantic (with no survivors), and their protracted and ultimately successful search for the two black boxes contained in that aircraft, planted the seed in my mind for the creation of this exceedingly informative, yet simple test of any state's healthcare regulatory system.

My first "brilliant idea" for how a state, any state, could better recognize the flaws in their current healthcare delivery system involves a comparison between two existing state regulatory agencies in South Carolina. I first presented this simple idea to my state representative, at that time the House assistant majority leader and a young (to me) attorney who I liked and respected very much. I assumed he would be able to see the logic in this simple idea.

Unfortunately such was not case. Within this book, I have the opportunity for a broad scope assessment of what I feel this simple test offers to any state's leadership strong enough to consider it.

First Step toward a State Regulatory Agency

Consider the tactics of Mothers Against Drunk Driving (MADD)—a well-recognized force in most state legislatures. Over the years they have found a way to compel state legislators to hear them and react favorably to their wishes. Such was the case in South Carolina several years ago that led to legislative changes regarding the DUI regulatory mechanism that eventually resulted in positive improvement in that state's drunk driving statistics. This positive step was so desperately needed (though much more needs to be done).

I offer a simple diagram of the point I am seeking to make.

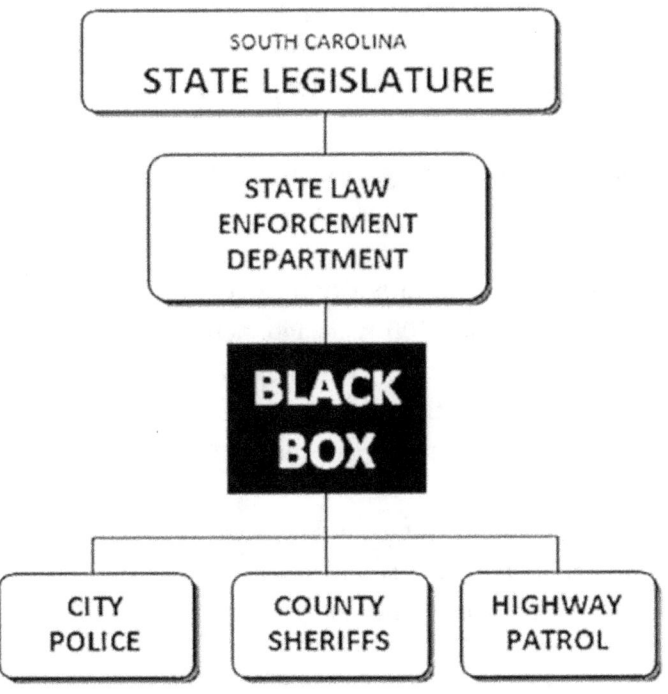

Next Step

In 1947, at the request of the South Carolina sheriffs, Governor Strom Thurman established by executive order the State Law Enforcement

Department (SLED). This department was created to provide assistance to all law enforcement agencies and allowed to delegate authority, through a regulatory mechanism, to the city police, county sheriffs, and the state highway patrol (the three recognized local agencies also mandated to regulate drunk-driving violations).

South Carolina's highest level of AUTHORITY created a state agency with authority sufficient to further delegate authority to local agencies—each of which had been created to provide ACCOUNTABILITY within their designated areas. However, that process of DELEGATING AUTHORITY to the local level required the presence of an intermediary regulatory mechanism, which I have euphemistically placed in a BLACK BOX. South Carolina legislators were later able to assess the benefit of their legislative improvements in their state's DUI regulations by revealing the results obtained from those three local law enforcement agencies throughout the state.

ORGANIZATIONAL STRUCTURE
+ AUTHORITY
+ DELEGATED AUTHORITY
= ACCOUNTABILITY

Who would have believed? Those prone to negativism will instantly jump to the fact that, "It's not perfect!" Well, no regulatory process run by humans will ever run perfectly; but it's better than what anyone might find in most parts of the world, and at least as good as other countries who try to do the same.

Let's now compare the regulatory mechanism that made a difference with DUI regulation to that assumed regulatory mechanism within the South Carolina healthcare delivery system.

South Carolina's highest level of authority created a State Board of Medical Examiners, as did every other state, more than 100 years ago. Some states (Alaska, Arizona, Hawaii, and New Mexico) had medical examiner boards even before they became states. The South Carolina State Board of Medical Examiners, like every other state board of medical examiners, was mandated to regulate the practice of medicine as provided by physicians within that state's borders.

A similar process (that was noted for the regulatory efforts involving drunk driving) is necessary for similar regulatory efforts regarding the practice of medicine. Figure 2 depicts the South Carolina regulatory mechanism for the practice of medicine. The State Board of

Medical Examiners is assumed to have been provided with sufficient authority to delegate authority through a regulatory mechanism to the LOCAL LEVEL of medical patient care.

Remember: All medical care is local. If you license them, you are obligated to regulate them!

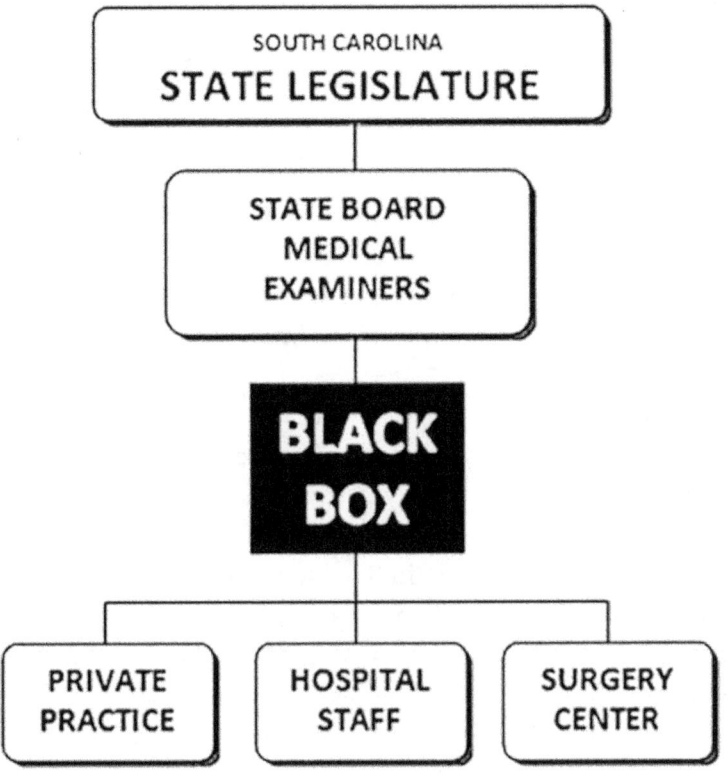

Fig. 2 Medical Regulatory Mechanism

FIND the Black Box containing the Medical Regulatory Mechanism

The primary component of each state's board of medical examiners is to "regulate the practice of medicine." Therefore one can presume that each state's board is where one should look for that state's *medical regulatory mechanism*. But don't be surprised if each state's board of medical examiners has difficulty producing such a *mechanism*.

In fact, hospitals (and surgery centers) are the ONLY places in America where an accidental death receives NO immediate review by a STATE SOURCE OF AUTHORITY.

Stop and think about that. An estimated twenty Boeing 747 airliners going down each week in our nation's hospitals—and no one in any state can FIND their state's medical regulatory mechanism? And none of the army of quality of healthcare experts has seemed to notice. The exercise of any state's efforts to find their Black Box might prove comical except for the fact that so many people are needlessly dying in their hospitals.

How to demand this First Step

Those who have lost a loved one to a needless hospital death can take a page from the MADD playbook, and come together under one umbrella, and with one purpose. Collectively confront your state legislature and demand that they replicate their efforts in the past for MADD, and now find (identify) their state's medical regulatory mechanism. Any effort to find the medical regulatory black box should bring them to the next demand.

Second Step

The best and quickest way to find out "Why Have We Not Gotten Further?," and why "Even if you cured cancer you couldn't get it to the people, because the medical system is broken," is to demand that some source of state authority begin to immediately track who responds, and how they respond, to the next needless hospital death in their state's healthcare delivery system.

People may be surprised, but shouldn't be, that no one in any state healthcare agency even hears about such tragic events until well after the fact, if at all. To find out how bad each state's healthcare delivery system truly is, try to track the response to a needless hospital death within your healthcare delivery system. Good luck!

The first and second steps go hand in hand to demonstrate how each and every state's healthcare delivery system is truly broken and how every governor and state legislator, past and present, have always been clueless regarding one of the most important components of their state's efforts to provide for their citizens.

Take special note of the sources that choose to speak against these tests and their potential for providing need-to-know information of a critical nature. Theoretically, every state governor and legislator should want to know, in detail, how their current healthcare delivery system functions. In reality, most governors and legislators would actually prefer not knowing, and just continue kicking that can down the road. (If you license them, you are obligated to regulate them!)

Third Step

This third step is offered to demonstrate how the army of quality of healthcare experts has completely failed in recognizing each state's responsibility regarding the healthcare delivery system.

There are reported to be forty-seven accredited schools of public health and seven associate schools. I assert that not one school of public health can be found to have a department head, or faculty member, who has written and taught on those two fundamentals of healthcare: that all medical care is local and states license doctors, therefore, states are responsible for the creation and maintenance of an effective healthcare delivery system. If my assertion were even only marginally true, this still illustrates the failure to recognize each state's responsibility in healthcare.

Now back to Dr. Elizabeth McGlynn, from the Rand Corporation, who said in 2004, "Only a fundamental redesign of the health system will improve the situation."

The major premise of *Find the Black Box* mirrors Dr. McGlynn's judgment of the situation except for one point: "redesign" assumes there is sufficient organizational structure in the current system to start with to allow for rearranging of the parts. The only way to save the healthcare delivery system at this point is to finally, and FOR THE FIRST TIME, begin to create a healthcare delivery system that recognizes the state's responsibility to create and maintain such a system.

Despite Machiavelli's view that there is nothing more difficult than attempting to create a new system, healthcare is important enough to attempt the *almost* impossible. Surely the nation that allowed men to walk on the moon and return them safely can assemble the expertise to create a healthcare delivery system based upon each state's responsibility. I offer a plan that goes far beyond anything ever imagined in this regard, but more on that later.

First Obstacle

Find the Black Box is predicated on the seemingly undeniable fact that states bear the major responsibility for the creation and maintenance of their state's healthcare delivery system—and—chaos will continue to reign in that aspect of healthcare until and unless that *fact* is recognized and dealt with in a meaningful manner.

The initial obstacle in redirecting all considerations for healthcare delivery system change is how to clarify and overcome the overwhelming focus on controlling the cost and access of healthcare—as if that would eliminate many, if not most, of our current healthcare problems. Sadly, nothing could be further from the truth. It is time to confront this first obstacle.

Two Aspects of Healthcare

In every discussion or conversation I've engaged in regarding healthcare during the years since writing two books about our healthcare delivery system, it took only moments for the other person to turn the subject to how to pay for healthcare after the fact.

Cost and access issues are vitally important and clearly in great need of increased understanding that would hopefully lead to beneficial change in each. However, even a perfect solution there, if possible, would still leave our nation with a broken healthcare delivery system. The "decision makers" don't get that.

I am convinced that I cannot repeat that point often enough to make people realize that the healthcare delivery system is just as important, and just as messed up, as how to pay for healthcare after the fact. They are each different aspects of the system as a whole, and each much be dealt with separately. These two vital aspects of our current healthcare system *must* be dealt with in complete isolation, one from the other.

Regina Herzlinger, in her book *Who Killed Healthcare?*, wrote that due to her three decades as a researcher and teacher, "I know the current system from top to bottom." She knows the cost and access aspects of healthcare and is fully qualified to participate and contribute in efforts to improve those issues. But Professor Herzlinger, I say with the utmost courtesy and respect, doesn't know beans about the healthcare delivery system issues.

Find the Black Box offers my expertise regarding the healthcare delivery system itself—that is what I know how to correct. I am as unqualified to contribute to efforts regarding cost and access issues as Professor Herzlinger is in dealing with delivery system issues.

I have attempted to articulate my point that the healthcare delivery system is a state responsibility (and is how and where patients enter the healthcare system) in every way I can think of to drive home this point. The *Wall Street Journal* printed two letters to the editors, offering my comments regarding RomneyCare:

"States Must Lead Health Reform," *Wall Street Journal.*
November 14, 2011

Regarding your editorial "Romney's Fiscal Awakening" (Nov. 8): You should examine in detail "RomneyCare Original," prior to its being legislatively compromised into "RomneyCare Modified." Next, ponder Newt Gingrich's sage advice contained in his 2010 Foreword for Governor Rick Perry's book *Fed Up*: "States have been called laboratories in democracy precisely because every problem potentially has fifty different approaches to solving it. Some solutions work in some states and not in others."

Finally, consider which offered our nation the more beneficial attempt to address the cost and access aspects of healthcare: RomneyCare Original in one state, ObamaCare poured over the entire nation by a democratically controlled Congress, or the far more usual response of doing nothing?

There are two basic fundamentals of healthcare that are constantly ignored: All medical care is local, and states license doctors to practice medicine. It is in the states where the reorganization of our highly dysfunctional healthcare system must begin. The federal government, with the best of intentions, is focusing on how to pay for care after the fact, and prevents the states from considering radical changes in the design of the healthcare system itself.

"RomneyCare 2.0 and Chances for a Reformed System," *Wall Street Journal,*
Aug. 15, 2012

RomneyCare "original" was twice modified, first by Gov. Mitt Romney's Democratic-led legislature and further modified by his succeeding governor and legislature. Furthermore, constant bashing of Gov. Romney's attempt to confront a major fiscal problem in his state gives left-handed praise to those forty-nine governors who chose to ignore the same problem in their states. Six years later, it is abundantly clear that there was not then, and there continues to be no perfect solution and no magic wand for that aspect of our healthcare system. Incremental change, preferably within one state at a time, was and continues to be a more prudent, test-tube type method for future efforts in confronting this health and fiscal disaster. Remember, as noted on the same page as this editorial, welfare change began in one state and was initiated by a Republican governor.

How to pay for healthcare and the healthcare delivery system are the two equally important, but completely different, aspects of our healthcare system. Our nation's priorities for healthcare change are being misdirected by the failure to give equal consideration for both the quality and cost of healthcare.

The constant criticism of Governor Romney's efforts has not been beneficial for the prospect of finding the next governor who might confront our dysfunctional healthcare delivery system.

Two Healthcare Imperatives

1. States are responsible for the healthcare delivery system.
2. Confront the two aspects separately and in isolation, one from the other.

The army of quality healthcare experts is so vast and diverse that no person could possibly name every agency, group, organization, foundation, think tank, school of public health, professional organizations, etc., currently seeking to "improve the quality of healthcare." But I will take a stab at doing just that in Chapter 3.

The fact that every state created a medical examining board over 100 years ago has to have some significance. Yet governors and state legislators, past and present, remain clueless regarding their states' responsibility for their states' healthcare delivery system. Where have these healthcare experts been?

I thought I had a sound understanding of our healthcare delivery system after writing my first book, *First, Do No Harm: The Cure for Medical Malpractice* (2004). That book received some positive reviews, including one from the *New England Journal of Medicine*.

Later, I thought I really understood that system far better after writing my second book, *Misdiagnosed! Why Current Healthcare Change is Malpractice* released in June 2010 with little notice, but something else, just as important to me was also taking place. In that book, I recognized the need for and the existing void regarding an organizational structure with clearly defined points of authority, responsibility, and accountability. I contend that that book contains more facts about the flaws in our current healthcare delivery system than any other two or three books combined out there. To my knowledge, no one has ever questioned the facts in any aspect of either of my books.

But several additional steps were still needed in order to pull all the parts together. This period of my increased understanding began in mid- 2010. I will share my process.

The Process

South Carolina House member Nikki Haley joined three other Republican candidates seeking to become the next governor in 2010. I was strongly leaning toward casting my lone vote for one of the other candidates when Nikki Haley said two things: "I will think outside the box," and "I will meet with any person who can contribute to making South Carolina better." The wheels in my mind began to turn. What would I tell a governor who says she will *listen*, and will *think outside the box*?

Thinking outside the box is like saying you plan to run a marathon, and then doing it. Each is easier said than done (I've done both). To think outside the box requires formulating a unique or highly different process, and then making it a reality. I thought outside the box over forty years ago in 1969–70 by creating the first mini-residency ever accomplished in any major surgical specialty in our healthcare system in Madison, Wisconsin. The second oral surgery mini-residency occurred at Parkland Hospital in Dallas, Texas, one or two years later; and the third was in their sister residency program in Fort Worth. Several other oral surgery residency programs soon followed suit.

The American Board of Obstetrics and Gynecology, in an article in 2003 on their volunteer peer review program of hospital departments of their specialty, were decrying their lack of mini-residencies. When I first read that article while researching the medical literature for my first book, I laughed and said to myself, "I did one of those thirty-three years ago."

But back to Governor Haley . . . .

The pieces necessary to think outside the healthcare box fell into place rapidly. I suddenly realized I could clearly see how to accomplish one of the most important and desperately needed feats in the history of our healthcare system. I became very excited because the entire process I could visualize was both logical and doable—if one could find a state governor who would listen to all of the details and give me and my outside-the-box process sincere consideration.

First, I will describe how to accomplish this most important healthcare feat; then I will describe why Governor Haley was not able to accept my offer. And also why, in the coming months, all of the South Carolina legislators that I met with came to the same unfortunate conclusion. Yet neither the governor nor any of those State legislators could deny, as stated by Dr. Taylor in his 2010 public acknowledgment, "The medical system is broken!"

Three-Phase Process to Completely Reorganize Healthcare

I first identified components that contribute to the current South Carolina healthcare delivery system:

State agencies:
Medical Examining Board
Department of Health and Environmental Control Department of Health and Human Services—and associated organizations:
  Medicare certification of hospitals: The Joint Commission
  DNV Healthcare, Inc.
  Quality Improvement Organization (Medicare certification)
  Quality Improvement Organization (Medicaid certification)
  Associations/Membership organizations:
    South Carolina Medical Association
    South Carolina Hospital Association
    Quality Improvement Organization (Medicare certification)
    Quality Improvement Organization (Medicaid certification)
  Associations/Membership organizations:
    South Carolina Medical Association
    South Carolina Hospital Association
  Arnold School of Public Health
  Moore School of Business
  Health Sciences of South Carolina
    Quality Improvement Council
  South Carolina Governor's Quality Award (Baldrige)

1. "Where are we now? and how did we get here?"

Qualified people (i.e. me/my staff) can act as agents behalf of the governor and legislature and meet with leaders from each component to engage in a *fact-finding process* (with emphasis on this not being a "gotcha" process), exploring:

What do you do? How do you do it? What can't you do?
What would you like to be able to do? etc.

Over the course of my medical career, I have given dozens of surgical malpractice legal depositions (fact-finding processes taken under oath).

The healthcare fact-finding process would be carried out just like a legal deposition, except the information would be obtained under the delegated authority provided by the governor and legislature.

Each of the healthcare leaders would be shown the list of the other components and asked, "Are we missing any healthcare component not listed?" to assure as complete and inclusive a process as possible—keeping in mind that such a process has never been done before (thinking outside the box).

The governor and legislature would then be provided with a complete, detailed picture of their state's current healthcare delivery system and how those components function, individually and collectively. Thus South Carolina, or the first state to accomplish this feat of thinking outside the healthcare box, would become the role model for every other state.

Many talk about our healthcare delivery system, but no one can describe it. No one has ever before attempted to describe it. This process would!

Point of caution: Too many decision makers want to bypass "Where are we now and how did we get here?" and go immediately to, "How do we fix the system?" Only bad things happen when decision makers change a system they cannot first describe, in detail. Unfortunately, our nation and every state have a long history of sad examples of such hubris.

2. Assess the Current Healthcare Delivery System

Once the state's decision makers would be able to see a detailed picture of their current healthcare delivery system, the governor and legislative leadership would access this composite structure and understand the true nature of their current healthcare delivery system's ability to function— and then determine whether this depicts an *acceptable* healthcare delivery system. (Rest assured it will not!)

Phases 1 and 2 could be accomplished in a matter of months, not years, if, and only if, the governor and legislative leaders demanded and obtained full cooperation from every component, including those outside the state contributors.

3. Big Tent Phase

After Sputnik circled the planet, Washington went into a panic. President Kennedy, in 1961, set the goal of being the first nation to have a man walk on the moon. Thus they built a "big tent" and invited qualified experts to join in making that outside-the-box thinking become reality. And they did.

But keep in mind: the only nation to put a man on the moon and return him safely has still never created (big tent), or even attempted to create, an organizational structure for its healthcare delivery system. Go figure.

Any state governor and legislature that might seek to benefit from what would be accomplished in Phases 1 and 2 in their state could use a similar "big tent" for the process of creating a new, organized, and functional healthcare delivery system. If and when that time comes, I would request the opportunity to offer a plan for the complete reorganization of any state's healthcare delivery system. My plan goes far beyond anything anyone has ever imagined (more on that later).

Food for thought: When states establish a healthcare delivery system, for that *system* to function properly, the system must operate at the LOCAL level and at the doctor/patient interface *throughout* the state. Does anyone see the need for a clearly defined organizational structure?

Governor Haley kindly met with me in August 2011 and that led to my meeting with Department of Health and Human Services Director Tony Keck in November 2011. But ultimately Governor Haley informed me that governors are sometimes incapable of doing everything they would like to do. She did not have the authority to accept my offer to help reorganize the state's dysfunctional healthcare delivery system. My meetings with several legislators led to the same conclusion at their level.

Naturally, I was disappointed. There is no doubt in my mind that the three-phase process I briefly described here could be the most important healthcare event since the famous Flexner Report that established the foundation for medical education, first here in America and later in Western Europe (one hundred years ago). Our entire nation desperately needs one state governor and legislature to find a way to make that happen.

In mid-2010 I had convinced myself that if Governor Haley, or any other governor, could find a way for me to provide them with the results of this three-phase process the current national debate regarding healthcare change would be redirected. But there was still one more piece missing in my understanding.

The Final Piece in the Process

Unaccountable: What Hospitals Won't Tell You and How Transparency Can Revolutionize Healthcare by Marty Makary, MD, allowed me to finally see the critical role and importance of AUTHORITY. Presidents and governors do not have individual authority, or at least they are not meant to have individual authority. Our nation's leaders, both at federal and state levels, have never had a complete understanding of authority— theirs or others.

Again, what is the highest level of authority in our nation for the creation of regulatory agencies? President + Senate/House majorities = national authority. And similarly, governor + Senate/House majorities = state authority.

Governors and state legislatures must *combine* their limited authority(s) for any process of their state's healthcare delivery system to be reorganized. Authority and delegated authority, properly recognized and utilized, are the missing ingredients necessary to think outside the healthcare box and make healthcare reorganization a reality. Otherwise, we keep what we've got, and we can see every day what a monumental dysfunctional mess that is.

Once it became clear to me that Governor Haley did not possess the ability to allow me to help her make our state's healthcare delivery system better, I began to meet with members of the legislature. Those meetings were no more fruitful, and for the same reason(s).

I found one aspect of their inability to give more than passive interest in my offer troubling—due to the following: Dr. Taylor's quote that the medical system is broken was published in April 2010, just before Candidate Haley got my wheels turning. And in April 2011 the chief administrator of Spartanburg Medical Center and past president of the South Carolina Hospital Association also publicly acknowledged in an article written by him reaffirming that "our healthcare system is broken."

A South Carolina senator with over thirty years in the senate and long-time chairman of the Senate Medical Affairs Committee was kind enough to speak with me by phone. I made him aware of the two public acknowledgements regarding our "broken" healthcare system by unimpeachable sources and of my interest and ability to assist in addressing that problem. He closed our brief, but congenial conversation with, "Good luck."

That South Carolina Senate leader was dismissively telling the people of South Carolina, "Good luck with your broken healthcare system."

No one disputes that our healthcare system is 'broken," yet the decision makers appear to be incapable of recognizing that fact and responding appropriately. What will it take for leaders to do more than PASSIVELY acknowledging that, "yes," they know the system is broken—AND—that they will DO SOMETHING about that fact?

60 Minutes helped to provide further insight in their segment, "Hospitals: The cost of admission," which aired on December 2, 2012. The target of that segment was Health Management Associates, Inc. (HMA). HMA operates about seventy hospitals, primarily in rural areas, in fifteen states. Former HMA employees, three ER physicians and one administrator, alleged that physicians were being pressured into admitting patients without need for admission, and such unnecessarily admitted patients were then put through a battery of tests, many of those tests, again, being medically unnecessary. In short, those four whistle-blowers were claiming that HMA was "ringing the cash register" without proper medical cause. An HMA spokesperson, naturally, denied the allegations.

I cite this example, not with the intent to determine the truth in this matter of alleged medical fraud, but to illustrate an overarching piece I see as sorely missing. No one mentioned the states' responsibility in this, or similar matters. HMA happens to have two HMA hospitals and seventeen HMA outpatient clinics in rural areas of South Carolina, and the state has three healthcare agencies: Medical Examining Board, Department of Health and Environmental Control (DHEC), and the Department of Health and Human Services (DHHS). Those three STATE agencies are (supposedly) assisted in the efforts to improve healthcare in the state by The Joint Commission, DNV-HC, and contracts with two quality improvement organizations.

I hear those who support the idea of state's rights and complain about how the federal government has wrongly assumed control over too many aspects of our economy and our lives—and how much of that control must be returned to the states. Theoretically, I'd agree, but reality tempers my ardor because state governors and state legislators, past and present, give no evidence that they could or ever will try to assume more responsibilities. They first need to demonstrate their ability to recognize their current responsibilities. Do those complainers demand more healthcare delivery system accountability from their states?

Then Candidate Haley led me to formulate the three-phase process for how any state can finally see a complete picture of their current system, and thereby hopefully assist those state leaders in recognizing the desperate need to reorganize. I have been convinced in recent years that I see something that no one else has ever seen before—and that it could be invaluable to making healthcare in America better. But Governor Haley and the state legislators I met with were unable or unwilling to try to find a way to make it happen. I am so tired of hearing what they CAN'T do. I am waiting for someone to say, "Let's make this happen because the need is so great, and too many people are dying needlessly in our hospitals."

Dr. Makary's book, *Unaccountable,* provided the clue that finally made all of the pieces fit together (authority, delegated authority, and organizational structure). If any governor and state legislature truly wants to make their state's healthcare delivery system better, they must recognize the importance of those three terms and their interrelationship.

Using South Carolina as an example, if any governor and state legislature ever combined their individual authorities to create a process that will provide them with complete details on how each component of their current healthcare delivery system functions, they will see clearly why healthcare in America is so dysfunctional. Those healthcare components function as though they all speak a different language.

> "It must be remembered that there is nothing more difficult to plan, more doubtful of success, nor more dangerous to manage than the creation of a new system. For the initiator has the enmity of all who would profit by the preservation of the old institutions and merely lukewarm defenders in those who gain by the new ones."
>
> ~ Niccolo Machiavelli

In spite of Machiavelli's many wise prophesies, *Find the Black Box* is intended to present a compelling case for truly thinking outside the box regarding healthcare change and make the delivery system a state (every state) responsibility that is embraced with vigor—as one might approach a LIFE AND DEATH SITUATION, because that is exactly the case.

The current model of our healthcare delivery system, if one can call it that, has never been *organized*. It has become so large and disorganized that it is impossible to integrate positive improvements throughout the entire "system" (a system with no systematic characteristics).

In presenting my arguments, I freely name names and give dates. However, I intend no malice nor question anyone's sincerity. I believe the subject, quality of healthcare, and the constantly increasing annual rate of needless hospital deaths clearly warrant hard questions to be asked and hopefully answered.

It never ceases to amaze me that our needless hospital death rate, the equivalent to several commercial airliner crashes each and every day, appears to fly under the governmental and media radar while so many smaller tragedies receive national press coverage. Perhaps it's the sheer size, plus the fact that it is spread throughout a system of more than 5,000 hospitals and a similar number of surgery centers in fifty states, that has led twenty-plus years of disgrace to be passively accepted.

Regardless of reason, our continuing needless hospital death rate deserves intense scrutiny—the entire healthcare delivery system of every state, including every doctor and dentist licensed to practice.

A point of interest regarding surgery centers: Oral surgeons established the national acceptance of surgery centers decades ago. Dr. Stuart Kelly began his oral surgery practice near the state capital in Madison, Wisconsin, in 1947. Shortly after opening his new practice, a small group of city leaders, including at least one physician, invited him to lunch.

When asked if he "put people to sleep" in his office, he replied, "Yes." He was told, "Well, we can't allow you to do that."

But Dr. Kelly continued to "put people to sleep" in his office across the street from the Wisconsin State Capitol. I joined Kelly, Griffin, and Linn in the practice of oral surgery in 1966. By 1980 that office had over 120 years of outpatient general anesthesia practice—with zero fatalities and no major anesthetic complications. President Kennedy's older sister,

Rosemary, was brought to our clinic on a regular basis for many years for her routine dental care under general anesthesia due to her inability to cooperate.

Now, I wonder: Does the estimate of over 5,000 surgery centers in the nation include oral surgery offices? And does anyone even know? It is impossible to "improve the system" without improving the entire system, including the surgery centers that no one talks about?

What's Still Missing?

The next chapter details what is missing, and has always been missing throughout our healthcare "system"—an inaccurate label for a very large, multi-component entity devoid of possessing even the slightest degree of functional "systematic" characteristics.

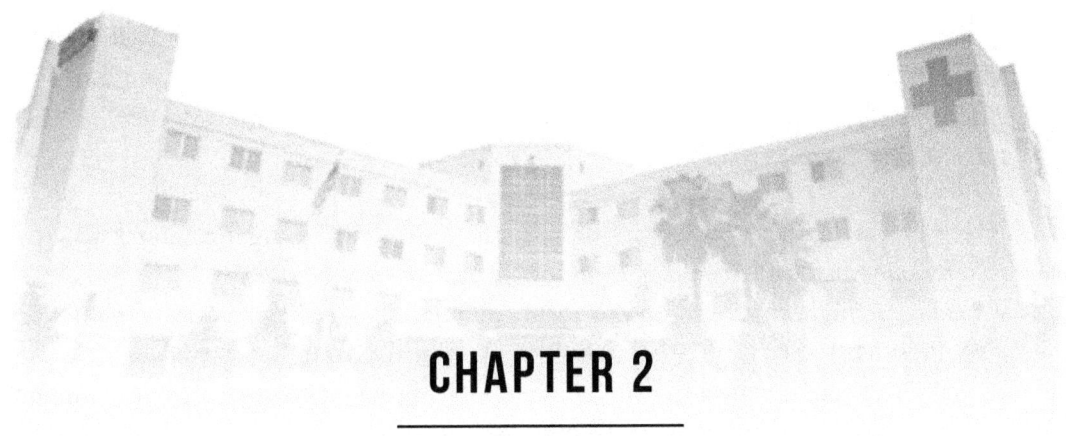

CHAPTER 2

WHAT'S MISSING?

ORGANIZATIONAL STRUCTURE is the typically hierarchical arrangement of lines of authority, communications, rights, and duties of an organization. Organizational structure determines how the roles, power, and responsibilities are assigned, controlled, and coordinated, and how information flows between the different levels of management.

ORGANIZATIONAL and **STRUCTURE** together are the first two of three key words that represent the most important elements that have always been missing in our healthcare delivery system. "Systems," to be effective, are multi-component collaborations with the intent directed toward cohesive function—characteristics found sorely lacking in our current healthcare system. Human bodies function normally due to the combined efforts of multiple multi-component *systems*. Where would we be without our bodily *systems*?

Test: Identify and describe the organizational structure of our current healthcare delivery system at any level of its entirety and within that portion of that system nearest you. Sadly, there is no structure there. Yet people continue to wonder how and why so many people can needlessly die within the greatest healthcare "system" ever allowed to exist.

Notice, I did not say the greatest healthcare "system" ever created.

The nation that allowed men to walk on the moon and return safely has never created, or even attempted to create, a healthcare delivery system with a clearly describable organizational structure. Our nation's healthcare system has evolved like a weed patch with no master gardener. The system that consumes almost 20 percent of the US economy has NO systematic characteristics, and never has had systematic characteristics.

Imagine Ford, General Electric, or any other large, multi-component enterprise seeking to function without an organizational structure. Impossible! But that is exactly what we expect from our nation's healthcare delivery system. Yet everyone, and I do mean everyone, has tolerated watching our healthcare delivery system muddle through crisis after crisis, and continually deteriorate before our eyes. Our nation has paid dearly in money and needlessly lives lost while decision makers, at every level, focused on other priorities. Look for the organizational structure of our current healthcare delivery system, and the more you search for what is not there, the more clearly you will see how chaotic and dysfunctional our current system truly is.

AUTHORITY is the third key word. But in its relationship to the organizational structure of a system, one must understand both *authority* and *delegated authority*.

What is the highest level of authority in our nation for the creation of regulatory agencies? President + Senate/House majorities. And in the same way, governor + Senate/House majorities equals state authority (except in Nebraska where they were wise enough to limit their state legislature to one collective house).

At each level of government, the three powers must combine their limited authorities in order to create (establish) systems (agencies). For example, all fifty states (and some even before becoming states) combined their powers within each state to separately create each of our fifty state boards of medical examiners over 100 years ago. Each state board is mandated to "regulate the practice of medicine" and thereby protect their citizens from negligent care. Unfortunately, none of the fifty state boards were created with a sufficiently defined organizational structure containing effective points of authority necessary to be able to fulfill that duty to their public. State medical examining boards have been some of the most ineffective aspects of our healthcare delivery system despite their long history of existence.

While large industries offer a convenient example of the need (absolute necessity) for an organizational structure, my personal experience with the benefits of having and functioning in such a system come from my twenty-three years of military service (four years of active duty in the US Air Force plus one additional month during the Cuban Crisis in 1962 and nineteen years combined in the Air Force Reserve, and in the Tennessee and Wisconsin Air National Guard and other sources of reserve activities).

A comparison of how I was delegated authority at my last active duty Air Force assignment in 1956 and allowed to utilize that delegated authority in performing my duties at that time illustrates what is missing and has always been missing within our healthcare delivery system. (My depiction of the US Air Force is intended to illustrate organizational structure, authority, and delegated authority in relation to my own tenure in the Air Force.)

US Air Force
Secretary of the Air Force Chief of Staff
Tactical Air Command Numbered Air Forces
5th Air Force (Korea and Japan) 1954–55 9th Air Force (US) 1955–57
461st Bombardment Wing, Tactical (TAC), Blytheville Air Force Base, Arkansas
Base/Wing Commander and Deputy Wing Commander
1st Lt. Ira Williams, Commander, Wing Headquarters Squadron

The organizational structure of the US Air Force delegated authority commensurate with an individual's level of responsibility. When I was transferred to the 461st Bombardment

Wing at Blytheville AFB, I assumed I would be assigned to one of the three bomb squadrons. Wrong! I suddenly found myself to be CO of the Wing Headquarters Squadron and a member of the Base/Wing Commander's Wing Staff, reporting directly to the Deputy Wing Commander. Shortly after, I was given an additional duty as the assistant trial counsel for summary court martial. My first appearance as such was before a summary court marital board consisting of two lieutenant colonels, three majors, four captains, and a first lieutenant. (I won the case.)

I was suddenly in charge of approximately 100 noncommissioned officers and enlisted men. Included in that group was one airman currently in the base stockade, awaiting an unscheduled thus far general court martial and requesting that his commander release him to the confines of the base until that trial was to take place.

Problem: No one, including our Wing Staff Judge Advocate, could determine if that airman's "commander" was the Base/Wing Commander or little old 1st Lt. Ira Williams. On 5 September 1956, 1st Lt. Ira Williams, Commander, signed the release order for Airman Puckett, and since no other Wing Staff officer would allow him to work for them, he became my twenty-four-hour responsibility. I also had to strap a .45 to my hip, line up my men, and pay them in cash once a month. I testified at Airman Puckett's general court martial during the late afternoon and early evening the day before Thanksgiving 1956. I testified on his behalf that I had ordered his release in the hope that his conduct while awaiting trial might prove beneficial for his defense, and "he didn't run."

There is much more to my sudden exposure to the fundaments of organizational structure, authority, and delegated authority; but suffice it to say that I still have copies of my original orders for the above points of fact.

Because of my combined experiences in a position of delegated authority in the Air Force, and as a surgical provider in our healthcare delivery system that is sorely lacking in those fundamental necessities, I have come to recognize the following ACCOUNTABILITY EQUATION.

AUTHORITY + RESPONSIBILITY = ACCOUNTABILITY
DELEGATED AUTHORITY + RESPONSIBILITY = ACCOUNTABILITY

But the ACCOUNTABILITY EQUATION, to be as effective as it can be and for meaningful accountability to take place, requires a clearly defined organizational structure with specific points of authority and delegated authority.

Accountability is a By-product of Authority!

ACCOUNTABILITY, the word, is replete in the quality of healthcare literature, while AUTHORITY, in the full recognition of its purpose and use, goes unnoticed. Yet, accountability can only become real and effective through the efforts of recognized authority, including delegated authority. Thus the paradox of our healthcare delivery system begins to be revealed.

Misdiagnosed! Why Current Healthcare Change is Malpractice is probably the first rudimentary attempt to diagram the organizational structure of our current healthcare delivery system. However, when I wrote that book, I had still not fully recognized the importance of the authority equation. All of that changed on Saturday, September 22, 2012, when I opened my *Wall Street Journal* and saw the front page article in Section C: *Unaccountable: What Hospitals Won't Tell You and How Transparency Can Revolutionize Healthcare* by Marty Makary, MD.

I read the article before 8:00 a.m. and had purchased a copy of the book from Barnes and Noble by 10:00 a.m. By Sunday, I had his book highlighted and underlined, and printed out a few quotes graciously permitted by Dr. Makary that struck a chord with me.

"I enrolled in the Harvard School of Public Health, where I discovered a great passion. I love studying the global burden of disease, ranking health priorities, and talking about how to change behaviors on a large scale."

"I am witnessing a generation eager to get at the root cause of our fragmented and uncoordinated system of care."

"Some hospitals and even individual doctors are taking a simple transparency pledge to participate in public reporting of outcomes, disclose all conflicts of interest, streamline patient access to records, and disclose mistakes as soon as they learn about them. I have taken this pledge, and I've posted it on the website for this book, unaccountablebook.com."

Less than two weeks later, Laura Landro, a *Wall Street Journal* healthcare staff writer, wrote a Bookshelf review of Dr. Makary's book and the following is the closing paragraph of her review:

"In addition to pushing for transparency, Dr. Makary argues that the "safety culture" of medicine must be improved. In the hierarchy of healthcare, doctors rule, and nurses and technicians are afraid to challenge them. That fear leads to the poor coordination of care and fear of reprisals for things like calling time out on a surgery if something seems amiss. In one recent Hopkins survey, employees at sixty reputable US hospitals were asked: "Would you feel comfortable receiving medical care in the unit in which you work?" At over half the hospitals surveyed, the answer was no."

It appears to me that Dr. Makary's book, *Unaccountable,* and Ms. Landro's critique might be, without either of them knowing it, recognizing that some fundamental need in our current healthcare delivery system is missing, but they don't quite know exactly what that something is. But one very important piece of evidence crops up in Ms. Landro's article: Quality of healthcare experts, including Dr. Makary, speak often of their strong desire to change and improve the "safety culture" in our healthcare delivery system.

Changing the "safety culture" in our healthcare system has become one of the consistent buzzwords within the quality of healthcare army of experts. I find the term similar to current attempts to reduce the incidence of obesity and the scourge of adult type 2 diabetes.

All three are highly laudable endeavors, but each can only become successful through individual behavioral modification on an enormous scale. Attempts to "change the safety culture" in our healthcare delivery system is one of those "generalities" that only a negative-obsessed person could possibly speak against. Yet with positive intent, I view "changing the safety culture" as just one more feel-good sound bite devoid of any means to judge the hoped-for result.

Since the *Wall Street Journal* was kind enough to print several of my letters to the editors in the past, Ms. Landro's review led me to write and submit my critique of Dr. Makary's book, which I consider a very positive step in the right direction:

> ***The Missing Link in Meaningful Healthcare Change***
>
> Both our federal and every state government have collectively poured trillions of dollars into a "system" no one can describe or has ever attempted to describe in detail. Healthcare consumes almost 20 percent of our national economy, directly impacts every living person, plus those yet unborn; and no one has a clue as to who has full authority and commensurate responsibility at any level of that so-called system. To make matters worse, if that's possible, no one can differentiate between federal and state authority and responsibility at most points within our current system.
>
> A simple test would suffice to illustrate the current healthcare delivery system dilemma. Search for the organizational structure and points of authority in both the national healthcare system and in each of the fifty states' systems. A "system" devoid of a clearly defined organizational structure, and lacking specific points of authority throughout its various components, is a "system" in name only.
>
> Authority must be present in order to provide accountability, but authority cannot exist and be delegated throughout the various levels of a "system" where there is no organizational structure. This fundamental dilemma replicates the old causality dilemma: Which came first, the chicken or the egg?
>
> We continue to pour billions of dollars into a system that is a non-system and into a system of quality of healthcare experts who have never recognized either the absence of, or the need for, an organizational structure with clearly defined points of authority, responsibility, and accountability. Every state created their state's medical examining board over 100 years ago. Yet every state governor and legislature since has ignored their responsibility to their citizens because of the dual facts that all medical care is local, and each state licenses its doctors to practice medicine within their state's unorganized "system."
>
> In his book released September 2012, titled *Unaccountable*, Marty Makary, MD, offers a perfect tool for demonstrating the dysfunction evident throughout our current healthcare system, while illustrating the predictable consequences that result from relying on a non-system that is devoid of an organizational structure and without sufficient self-contained authority to enable meaningful accountability to function throughout that "system."

Wall Street Journal did not see fit to print my letter.

Food for Thought

South Carolina has sixty-five hospitals and sixty-eight surgery centers located in all parts of the state. The challenge I propose: Find the points of functional authority and delegated authority in the SC healthcare delivery system. (I can't, and I've looked.)

Accountability is a by-product of authority. Those who focus on accountability in healthcare while ignoring the primary function of and need for CLEARLY DEFINED POINTS OF AUTHORITY demonstrate their lack of understanding about why the rate of needless hospital deaths has been going in the wrong direction for the last two decades and continues to do so.

Dr. Makary has received national recognition and praise for transparently confronting major failings within our entire healthcare delivery system and for offering several "concrete measures for tracking hospital performance." In *Unaccountable*, he suggests, "Congress should make transparency a condition of Medicare reimbursement and other types of funding."

As one of the more recent members of an army of quality of healthcare experts to gain national recognition, Dr. Makary offers well-intended considerations for positive change within a "system." But the fatal flaw in his prescription is that there is no functioning "system" capable of implementing those improvements because there is a complete lack of said organizational structure. Dr. Makary mentions "accountability" almost two dozen times, but he never describes the mechanism by which such accountability might take place or under what authority. Dr. Makary's title says it all: *Unaccountable!*

Our nation's military services have performed as well as they have because they were provided with two characteristics necessary for success: an ORGANIZATIONAL STRUCTURE and the ability to DELEGATE AUTHORITY. Our nation's healthcare delivery system has never possessed either necessary characteristic.

Authority was necessary to create our various military services, and that authority could only become sufficiently potent for that task through the combined consent of the then president and both Houses of Congress. That combined constitutional authority permitted the creation of an organizational structure for each military service, and allowed each service to delegate further authority commensurate with their responsibility at various levels throughout their branch of service.

How many times has anyone familiar with the military heard, "Sergeants run the army"? Picture a military unit without *functional delegated authority*.

A close examination of how each component of our military services function at every level, both here and abroad, as compared to the rampant dysfunction throughout every component of our nation's healthcare delivery system, will demonstrate the functional benefit of a clearly defined organizational structure with specific points of authority, responsibility, and accountability at every level.

Attempts to improve the quality of care within our current, unorganized "system" will continue to be ineffective until our healthcare delivery systems at the state level are completely reorganized (make that finally organized). A logical and doable reorganization process is readily available for that task, but the need for such reorganization must be recognized first—at both the federal and state levels. Such recognition would require state level decision makers to confront this critical issue in a new and different manner.

The missing link in meaningful healthcare change is the absence of AUTHORITY, properly DELEGATED throughout an equally important ORGANIZATIONAL STRUCTURE necessary for any "system" to function systematically.

I would like to ask Dr. Makary, and his conscientious colleagues who are signing his pledge for greater transparency, the same question I asked Dr. Wachter, here in Greenville in 2010: "How can you get your system into every hospital in the nation?" I am confident that Dr. Makary, like Dr. Wachter, is unable to answer that most important question.

Most healthcare in America takes place in hospitals throughout America, and not just in medical centers and teaching hospitals. More people are needlessly dying in our hospitals now than were over twenty years ago because all of the quality of healthcare "theoretical" improvements cannot become reality where the rubber meets the road due to the lack of an organizational structure that could permit such wide dissemination.

Now back to 1st Lt. Ira Williams, CO, Wing Headquarters Squadron. Blytheville AFB….

I spent more than a year as an aviation cadet prior to being commissioned as a second lieutenant at age twenty and receiving my navigator wings the year they welcomed the first class of cadets to the newly established Air Force Academy (1954). Some of my classmates resigned their new commissions and set aside their new wings in order to enter that first class. Some made it through, and some did not. Cadets become well versed in cleaning toilets, waxing floors, and walking tours in full dress uniform with white gloves in the hot Texas sun if they had accumulated sufficient demerits, often coming from white-gloved inspections of our living quarters (I speak from experience).

My delegated authority was primarily over those enlisted personnel who worked in Wing Headquarters and lived in a barracks on base. One day, early in my new position of authority, I walked through the barracks assigned to my men and was not pleased with what I saw. I contacted several of the senior noncommissioned officers who lived in that barracks and told them to pass the word to everyone: "All Wing Headquarters Squadron enlisted personnel are restricted to the base until their living quarters pass my inspection, and I have notified the Air Police at the main gate of my order." The Wing Headquarters Squadron barracks living quarters stopped looking like a college frat house in short order.

Find a hospital anywhere in America that can demonstrate medical staff individuals with delegated authority, plus evidence of the use of that authority by taking responsibility for providing accountability. Every hospital medical staff has chiefs of surgery, radiology, pathology, etc., but I doubt if anyone can find any evidence of accountability consistently used by such authority where and when it is most needed. Later I will share an excellent example of such a failure to utilize hospital medical staff authority. Actually, Dr. Robert Wachter will provide that example through his regularly scheduled discussions via the Agency for Healthcare Research and Quality (AHRQ) *WebM&M* morbidity and mortality rounds on the web. All too often what they don't say is more important than what they do say, if, and only if, one can recognize the importance of what they don't say.

Side Note: I am not attempting to use Dr. Wachter as a foil. I believe when a person, "yours truly" included, writes a nonfiction book or permits someone to introduce them as one of the world's premier experts on the quality of patient care, as Dr. Wachter was introduced here in Greenville SC, that person can (must) be judged by what they say and write. The dysfunction in our healthcare delivery system should be given the highest priority, and everyone who has been taking credit for their efforts to improve that system should be called upon to answer why there is scant evidence of improvement throughout that system.

Dr. Makary's book *Unaccountable* courageously peeks behind the curtain of our healthcare delivery system and shines a light on many of the problems long inherent in that system, but Find The Black Box speaks to both the Problems and the Solution.

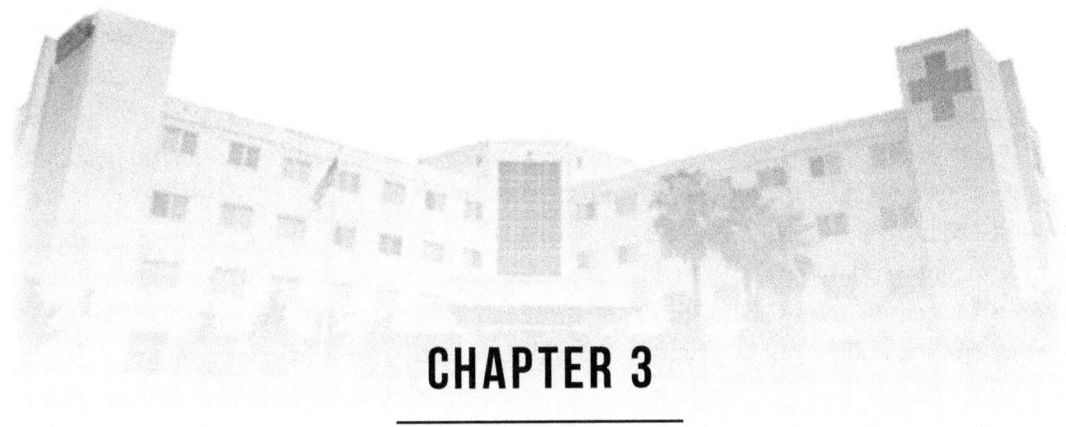

CHAPTER 3

QUALITY OF HEALTHCARE ARMY OF EXPERTS

No one can deny that our healthcare system has problems in every direction one might look. But the current primary focus on how to pay for healthcare after the fact, while the estimated needless hospital death rate is going in the wrong direction, is, to say the least, misguided. BOTH aspects are equally important.

The 1990 Harvard School of Public Health estimate of 98,000 needless hospital deaths annually was the first research project of its kind, particularly due to the four years spent in accumulating that understanding. The magnitude of the researchers' estimate was met with mixed reviews, particularly from the components of organized medicine. But no one could refute their findings; therefore, their estimate became the baseline used in *To Err Is Human*.

An army of quality of healthcare experts began to take shape, and has now become so enormous and so widely diverse as to defy complete description, but I offer an abbreviated representative list here. Keep in mind that, as that army of quality of healthcare experts has grown—and continues to grow, so has the estimated annual rate of needless hospital deaths. Thus far I have provided reasons why the efforts of that army of quality of healthcare experts have been so "unproductive." Now I will provide specific examples of that army's efforts, and add my contrarian response. I include complete copies of some materials for two reasons: so you can see WHAT they say and HOW they say it, and so you can also read between their lines to see what they don't say.

Experts

The US Congress has three committees with subcommittees on health in the US Senate, and seven committees with subcommittees on health in the House of Representatives. Members of Congress have been armed with numerous staff member experts and supported by many lobbyist "friends" as they have produced an endless supply of healthcare "improvements," which I will refer to shortly.

Congressional subcommittees, however, are *not* a part of the quality of healthcare army of experts. Congressional subcommittees are more like the "patron saints" of the quality of healthcare army of experts. One only has to read, with discernment, the fifty-three recommendations contained in six of the *Crossing the Quality Chasm* series of seven books to see how many, if not most, of those recommendations seek increased *authority*, responsibility, and, of course, increased funding, in order to continue to make healthcare far safer in America. Most problematic is that congressional subcommittees rarely, if ever, check track records before continuing to support efforts that cry out for detailed review.

If you had a loved one die a needless hospital death, what do your state leaders owe you? As has been established: states license doctors and all medical care is local. But most of the efforts to improve the quality of healthcare are, and continue to be, created by experts with *no ties* to state government. As we see, state governmental leaders seem to have taken little, if any, interest in the fact that their state's healthcare delivery system is, and has long been, broken. (I would welcome a true debate on this last point.)

Compare and Contrast QHC Army of Experts in the US

This list of quality of healthcare experts should provide an understanding of how enormous this army of highly educated and highly dedicated individuals has been, and how they continue to grow. A review of their own literature will follow in an attempt to illustrate a quality of healthcare "chasm" between what their literature says, and what is taking place in the real world of our nation's healthcare delivery system.

~Department of Health and Human Services (DHHS)
    Office of Inspector General (OIG)
    Office of Evaluation and Inspection (OEI)
    Agency for Healthcare Research and Quality (AHRQ)
    Centers for Medicare and Medicaid (CMS)
National Academy of Science (NAS)
Institute of Medicine (IOM)
National Quality Forum (NQF): Over 400 member organizations (beginning with AMA). The most active contributors to the current efforts to improve the quality of healthcare are associated with NQF member organizations.
Organized Medicine (AMA, ACOP, ACOS, medical specialties, etc.)
    American College of Medical Quality
The Joint Commission (organized medicine creation, 1951) Institute for Healthcare Improvement (IHI) (Dr. Donald Berwick)
Healthcare journals and publications, i.e., *JAMA, NEJM, Health Affairs*, etc.
~Schools of Public Health in the US: 47 accredited/7 associate

~Kaiser Permanente, managed care consortiums, etc.
~Foundations, i.e. Duke, MacArthur, Robert Wood Johnson, etc.
~Multiple Think Tanks, i.e. Rand, Cato, Heritage, Manhattan Institute, etc. Leapfrog Group and other big business efforts to better control their cost of healthcare for their companies and their employees (Such groups have made extremely positive contributions.) Patient-Centered Outcomes Research Institute (PCORI) (My apologies to the numerous contributors unrecognized.)

Good news: There is, and long has been, an army of highly educated and highly dedicated quality of healthcare experts—organizations, agencies, and individuals seeking to improve the quality of healthcare in America.

Bad news: The methods used thus far by that army of experts deserve to be questioned based on the increase in the annual rate of needless hospital deaths. (Surgery centers are still not mentioned nor is there any discussion of each and every state's responsibility.)

When QHC experts set a clearly defined goal (i.e., *To Err Is Human* in 1999) to reduce the 1990 estimate of needless hospital deaths by 50 percent in five years, and more than ten years later the goal is still so far out of reach, prudent people would be seeking answers from any and every source.

QHC experts can only provide isolated examples of positive improvements in a few selected medical centers and teaching hospitals, but most healthcare occurs in local communities throughout America. South Carolina has sixty-five hospitals. I would like to have some QHC experts take me on a tour through several of the small community hospitals scattered throughout South Carolina (where the healthcare rubber meets the patient care road) and demonstrate how their highly touted quality of healthcare improvements have become reality.

A Limited History of the Evolution of QHC Army of Experts

Armies can only materialize over time, and such is the case with our current, enormous, and constantly growing quality of healthcare army of experts. Numerous professional and nonprofessional organizations had been seeking ways to make patient care safer in our nation's hospitals for many years; but slightly over two decades ago, a pair of questionable patient care studies became the catalyst for:

- The creation of several additional QHC organizations by the federal government, and a rapid expansion of their mandates and efforts.
- The creation of army of experts' QHC organizations (government and nongovernment) coalescing their efforts and eventually beginning to harmonize their messages, constantly protected by confirmation bias.

The Institute of Medicine, in *To Err Is Human,* is consistently cited as the place and time when a far more coordinated quest for greatly improved quality of healthcare originated, AND the evolution of a process began to merge widely diverse organizations into what has now become a quality of healthcare army of experts. Therefore *To Err Is Human* is where further consideration should begin.

To Err is Human

To Err Is Human: Building a Safer Health System, Institute of Medicine, November 1999 [first four paragraphs quoted here]

Healthcare in the United States is not as safe as it should be—and can be. At least 44,000 people, and perhaps as many as 98,000 people, die in hospitals each year as a result of medical errors that could have been prevented, according to estimates from two major studies. Even using the lower estimate, preventable medical errors in hospitals exceed attributable deaths to such feared threats as motor-vehicle wrecks, breast cancer, and AIDS.

Medical errors can be defined as the failure of a planned action to be completed as intended or the use of a wrong plan to achieve an aim. Among the problems that commonly occur during the course of providing healthcare are adverse drug events and improper transfusions, surgical injuries and wrong-site surgery, suicides, restraint-related injuries or death, falls, burns, pressure ulcers, and mistaken patient identities. High error rates with serious consequences are most likely to occur in intensive care units, operating rooms, and emergency departments.

Beyond their cost in human lives, preventable medical errors exact other significant tolls. They have been estimated to result in total costs (including the expense of additional care necessitated by the errors, lost income and household productivity, and disability) of between seventeen billion and twenty-nine billion dollars per year in hospitals nationwide. Errors also are costly in terms of loss of trust in the healthcare system by patients and diminished satisfaction by both patients and health professionals. Patients who experience a long hospital stay or disability as a result of errors pay with physical and psychological discomfort. Health professionals pay with loss of morale and frustration at not being able to provide the best care possible. Society bears the cost of errors as well, in terms of lost worker productivity, reduced school attendance by children, and lower levels of population health status.

A variety of factors have contributed to the nation's epidemic of medical errors. One oft-cited problem arises from the decentralized and fragmented nature of the healthcare delivery system—or "non-system," to some observers. When patients see multiple providers in different settings, none of whom has access to complete information, it becomes easier for things to go wrong. In addition, the processes by which health professionals are licensed and accredited have focused only limited attention on the prevention of medical errors, and even these minimal efforts have confronted resistance from some healthcare organizations and providers. Many providers also perceive the medical liability system as a serious impediment to systematic efforts to uncover and learn from errors. Exacerbating these problems, most third-party purchasers of healthcare provide little financial incentive for healthcare organizations and providers to improve safety and quality.

The four-year study in New York State hospitals in 1990 that estimated 98,000 needless hospital deaths annually was the number *To Err Is Human* used to base their prediction of a 50 percent reduction in five years. Unfortunately, as is clearly evident, the estimated annual needless hospital death rate is now far higher—equivalent to "twenty Boeing 747 crashing each week."

One of the observations made in *To Err Is Human*, but easily overlooked: "One oft-cited problem arises from the decentralized and fragmented nature of the healthcare delivery system—or 'non-system,' to some observers."

Even in 1999 some of the QHC experts were aware that our nation's healthcare delivery system was a *non-system,* but the same experts are still unable to recognize the full meaning of that word *system,* and that each state is responsible for their own state's healthcare delivery system.

Timeline Review

1996: Due to studies regarding the quality of healthcare, the Institute of Medicine (IOM) launched a concerted effort focused on assessing and improving the nation's quality of care.

1997: New developments:

- IOM studies which led to *To Err Is Human* (1999) and *Crossing the Quality Chasm* (2001)
- AMA created a new member for the QHC army: National Patient Safety Foundation (after abandoning their failed efforts to create special medical malpractice courts with federal government assistance)
- AMA House of Delegates passed the first of four parliamentary votes that led to the creation of the Litigation Center (See Chapter 5).

Timelines provide a more detailed perspective of the enormous efforts to improve the quality of healthcare in America, because other organizations, i.e. organized medicine, etc., were also making their attempts to "improve the quality of patient care" outside the growing spectrum of efforts by the QHC army.

Crossing the Quality Chasm Series

To Err Is Human became the first in a series of seven books that make up the IOM *Crossing the Quality Chasm Series*. I list here the six books of that series that I have reviewed. Those six books contain fifty-three recommendations.

To Err Is Human: Building a Safer Health System (2000) 9 recommendations.

Crossing the Quality Chasm: A New Health System for the 21st Century, (2001) 13 recommendations.

Leadership by Example: Coordinating Government Roles in Improving Healthcare Quality (2002) 8 recommendations.

Health Professions Education: A Bridge to Quality (2003) 10 recommendations.

Priority Areas for National Action: Transforming Healthcare Quality (2003) 6 recommendations.

Patient Safety: Achieving a New Standard for Care (2004) 7 recommendations.

A review of the fifty-three recommendations provides a glimpse of the early vision many of the QHC army of experts had, and still have, for improving the quality of healthcare. Those recommendations describe a theoretical world of centralized expertise offering grandiose prognostications of future quality of healthcare improvements that can only be achieved by their plan to introduce their efforts throughout the "decentralized and fragmented nature of the healthcare delivery system—or non-system," to some observers." So, they know what they want to do, but they don't know how to make their efforts become reality throughout the current system. Attempting to read those fifty-three recommendations, while trying to imagine how any of them can become reality in most hospitals throughout that huge system is difficult to do. One must also realize the enormous number of highly educated healthcare experts who collaborated over many months, and with much expense in order to accumulate this immense collection of what has proven to be theoretical nonsense in the real healthcare world. But IOM was only just beginning:

The Healthcare Imperatives: Lowering Costs and Improving Outcomes

Workshop Series Summary
The IOM Roundtable on Value and Science-driven Healthcare convened stakeholders from across the healthcare field in a series of four two-day meetings titled: "The Healthcare Imperative: Lowering Costs and Improving Outcomes 2010."

Core concepts and principles

For the purpose of the roundtable activities, we define science-driven healthcare broadly to mean that, to the greatest extent possible, the decisions that shape the health and healthcare of Americans—by patients, providers, payers, and policymakers alike—will be grounded on a reliable evidence base, will account appropriately for individual variation in patient needs, and will support the generation of new insights on clinical effectiveness. Evidence is generally considered to be information from clinical experience that has met some established test of validity, and the appropriate standard is determined according to the requirements of the intervention and clinical circumstance. Processes that involve the development and use of evidence should be accessible and transparent to all stakeholders.

A common commitment to certain principles and priorities guides the activities of the Roundtable and its members, including the commitment to: the right healthcare for each person; putting the best evidence into practice; establishing the extent effectiveness, efficiency, and safety of medical care delivered; building constant measurement into our healthcare investments; the establishment of healthcare data as a public good; shared responsibility distributed equitably across stakeholders, both public and private; collaborative stakeholder involvement in priority setting; transparency in the execution of activities and reporting of results; and subjugation of individual political or stakeholder perspectives in favor of the common good.

All I can say is, WOW!

The Workshop Series Summary (over 600 pages) listed four sections, containing twenty-two segments and over seventy presentations, and provided a glimpse into the enormous size and diversity of the current quality of healthcare army of experts. There appeared to be no mention of the state's (each state's) responsibility or of the question I asked Dr. Wachter in 2010: "How do you get these praise-worthy offerings to every hospital in America?"

The Institute of Medicine in *To Err Is Human* justifiably claims credit for utilizing the findings of two earlier research projects, one in Colorado and Utah, but most importantly, the four-year study in Upstate New York hospitals by Brennan and Leape that provided the estimated baseline of 98,000 needless hospital deaths annually. But this is also when the various governmental and nongovernmental organizations began to coalesce into the quality of healthcare army of experts of today.

Agency for Healthcare Research and Quality (AHRQ)

AHRQ is one of twelve agencies within the Department of Health and Human Services and is the lead agency charged with supporting research designed to improve the quality of healthcare, reduce its cost, improve patient safety, address medical errors, and broaden access to essential services. AHRQ sponsors and conducts research that provides evidence-based information on healthcare outcomes, quality, cost, use, and access. AHRQ was established in 1989 and its headquarters are in Rockville, Maryland.

Dr. Carolyn Clancy, AHRQ director, in her Performance Budget Submission for Congressional Justification for fiscal year 2008 stated, "We are seeing results of efforts to improve quality of care. AHRQ released the fourth annual reports focusing on quality of and disparities in healthcare in America. Overall, the review of forty core quality measures found a 3.1 percent increase in the quality of care—the same rate of improvement as the previous two years.

AHRQ headquarters is located in a standalone building surrounded by a large parking lot with hundreds of automobiles, a very high chain-link fence and security guards at the gate. On the morning of November 17, 2008, I paid an unscheduled visit to the AHRQ headquarters and was told by the guard that I had ten minutes in order to make a connection in the headquarters. He did not tell me what consequences I might face IF I failed to be successful. Fortunately I was successful in meeting with one of the administrative assistants for AHRQ Director Dr. Carolyn Clancy. My unscheduled visit was very timely because I learned that Dr. Clancy was attending a NQF National Priorities Partnership press announcement meeting scheduled for that afternoon in Washington DC that I was able to attend, but more on that huge event later.

AHRQ (formerly Agency for Healthcare Policy and Research) has been active in the efforts to improve the quality of healthcare in America for many years, as evident by a visit to their website, which I find overwhelming with information and repositories of patient care data. It would be impossible to describe the broad scope of AHRQ efforts regarding patient safety in detail, therefore this brief review will be limited to:

Evidence-Based Medicine (EBM) and Evidence-Based Practice (EBP)

What is evidence-Based Practice (EBP)(quoted from the web site)

> The most common definition of EBP is taken from Dr. David Sackett, a pioneer in evidence-based practice. EBP is "the conscientious, explicit, and judicious use of current best evidence in making decisions about the care of the individual patient. It means integrating individual clinical expertise with the best available external clinical evidence from systematic research." (Sackett D, 1996)
>
> EBP is the integration of clinical expertise, patient values, and the best research evidence into the decision making process for patient care. Clinical expertise refers to the clinician's culminated experience, education and clinical skills. The patient brings to the encounter his or her own personal and unique concerns, expectations, and values. The best evidence is usually found in clinically relevant research that has been conducted using sound methodology. (Sackett D, 2002)
>
> The evidence, by itself does not make a decision for you, but it can help support the patient care process. The full integration of these three components,

Clinical Expertise, Best Research Evidence, and Patient Values and Preferences, into clinical decisions enhances the opportunity for optimal clinical outcomes and quality of life. The practice of EBP is usually triggered by patient encounters which generate questions about the effects of therapy, the utility of diagnostic tests, the prognosis of disease, or the etiology of disorders.

Evidence-Based Practice requires new skills of the clinician, including efficient literature searching, and the application of formal rules of evidence in evaluating the clinical literature.

The Steps in the EBP Process

ASSESS the patient. 1. Start with the patient—a clinical problem or question arises from the care of the patient.

ASK the question. 2. Construct a well-built clinical question derived from the case.

ACQUIRE the evidence. 3. Select the appropriate resource(s) and conduct a search.

APPRAISE the evidence. 4. Appraise that evidence for its validity (closeness to the truth) and applicability (usefulness in clinical practice).

APPLY: talk with the patient. 5. Return to the patient— integrate that evidence with clinical expertise, patient preferences, and apply it to practice.

Self-Evaluation: 6. Evaluate your performance with the patient.

Evidence-Based Practice Centers

Synthesizing scientific evidence to improve quality and effectiveness in healthcare
[quoted from the web site]

Under the Evidence-based Practice Centers (EPC) Program of AHRQ, five-year contracts are awarded to institutions in the United States and Canada to serve as EPCs. The EPCs review all relevant scientific literature on clinical, behavioral, and organization and financing topics to produce evidence reports and technology assessments. These reports are used for informing and developing coverage decisions, quality measures, educational materials and tools, guidelines, and research agendas. The EPCs also conduct research on methodology of systematic reviews.

In 1997, AHRQ launched its initiative to promote evidence- based practice and everyday care through establishment of the Evidence-based Practice Center (EPC) Program. The EPCs develop evidence reports and technology assessments on topics relevant to clinical and other healthcare organization and delivery issues;—specifically those that are common, expensive, and are significant for the Medicare and Medicaid populations. With this program, AHRQ became a "science partner" with private and public organizations in their efforts to improve the quality, effectiveness, and appropriateness of healthcare by synthesizing the evidence and facilitating the translation of evidence-based research findings. Topics are nominated by non-federal partners such as professional societies, health plans, insurers, employers, and patient groups.

In August 2012 AHRQ announced the fourth award of five-year contracts for EPC-IV to eleven evidence-based practice centers to continue the work performed by the previous group of EPCs. Those EPCs chosen include ten institutions and organizations across the scope of the nation and one institution in Canada.

Report development

The EPCs review all relevant scientific literature on clinical, behavioral, and organization and financing topics to produce evidence reports, technical reviews (covering nonclinical methodological topics) and technology assessments.

These reports, reviews, and technology assessments are based on rigorous, comprehensive synthesis and analysis of the scientific literature on topics relevant to clinical, social science/ behavioral, economic, and other healthcare organization and delivery issues. EPC reports and assessments emphasize explicit and detailed documentation of methods, rationale, and assumptions. These scientific syntheses may include meta- analysis and cost analysis. All EPCs collaborate with other medical and research organizations so that a broad range of experts is included in the development profits.

The resulting evidence reports and technology assessments are used by Federal and State agencies, private sector professional societies, health delivery systems, providers, payers, and others committed to evidence-based healthcare.

Note: One can only assume that the work of the AHRQ EPC since 1997 allowed Dr. Clancy to announce in 2008: "Overall, the review of forty core quality measures found a 3.1 percent increase in the quality of care—the same rate of improvement as the previous two years."

AHRQ WebM&M

Morbidity & mortality rounds on the web

AHRQ *WebM&M*) is the peer-reviewed, web-based journal on patient safety. Funded by the Agency for Healthcare Research and Quality (AHRQ), the site is edited by Doctors Robert Wachter and Kaveh Shojania, along with a team at the University of California, San Francisco (UCSF), with technical support from DoctorQuality. The site is free and has no advertisements.

AHRQ *WebM&M* is designed to educate providers and trainees about patient safety and medical errors by using a case-based approach in an engaging, blame-free environment.

The 1999 report by the Institute of Medicine (IOM) *To Err is Human: Building a Safer Health System* created tremendous interest in improving patient safety. Every month in hospitals across the country, morbidity and mortality (M&M) conferences convene for discussion of specific cases that raise issues regarding medical errors and quality improvement. Although M&M conferences have been a staple at most American hospitals for decades, until now there has been no comparable national forum to discuss and learn from medical errors. AHRQ and the University of California, San Francisco, saw the opportunity to use the Web to host a national Morbidity and Mortality conference aimed at improving patient safety through analysis of anonymous cases. This concept evolved into the AHRQ *WebM&M* (morbidity and mortality) site.

One of several themes this book seeks to illustrate is how the quality of healthcare army of experts have coalesced under one exceedingly large umbrella where confirmation bias and harmonization seem to exclude the existence of contrarian considerations. Support for my characterization of this quality of healthcare army of experts, I believe, can be found by reviewing the enormous membership list of NQF and of the boards of directors, editorial boards and advisory panels that are listed with the other organizations. For instance, AHRQ *WebM&M* has seventeen members of its editorial board and thirty-five members of its advisory panel.

Dr. Paul A. Gluck, a professor in the Department of Obstetrics and Gynecology at the University of Miami Miller School of Medicine in Miami, Florida, is the author of the American College of Obstetrics and Gynecology article noted elsewhere in this book regarding their voluntary system of medical peer review that stated their specialty's great need for mini-residencies. Dr. Gluck is also a past chairman of the board of the National Patient Safety Foundation.

AHRQ *WebM&M* offers twenty-three Patient Safety Primers. A selected few provided here [as written on the site]

> Patient Safety Primers guide you through key concepts in patient safety. Each primer defines a topic, offers background information on its epidemiology and context, and highlights relevant content from both AHRQ PSNet and AHRQ *WebM&M*.
>
> **Adverse Events after Hospital Discharge.** Being discharged from the hospital can be dangerous for patients. Nearly 20 percent of patients experience an adverse event in the first three weeks after discharge, including medication errors, healthcare- associated infections, and procedural complications.
>
> **Diagnostic Errors.** Thousands of patients die every week due to diagnostic errors. While clinicians' cognitive biases play a role in many diagnostic errors, underlying healthcare system problems also contribute to missed and delayed diagnoses.

Disruptive and Unprofessional Behavior: Popular media often depicts physicians as brilliant, intimidating, and condescending in equal measures. This stereotype, though undoubtedly dramatic and even amusing, obscures the fact that disruptive and unprofessional behavior by clinicians poses a definite threat to patient safety.

Error Disclosure. Many victims of medical errors never learn of the mistake, because error is simply not disclosed. Physicians have traditionally shied away from discussing errors with patients, due to fear of precipitating a malpractice lawsuit and embarrassment and discomfort with the disclosure process.

Never Events. The list of never events has expanded over time to include adverse events that are unambiguous, serious, and usually preventable. While most are rare, when never events occur, they are devastating to patients and indicate serious underlying organizational safety problems.

Safety Culture: High-reliability organizations consistently minimize adverse events despite carrying out intrinsically hazardous work. Such organizations establish a culture of safety by maintaining a commitment to safety at all levels, from front-line providers to managers and executives.

AHRQ and NQF have been closely aligned since AHRQ began their Evidence-based Practice Centers in 1997. IOM had begun the research process that led to *To Err Is Human* in 1999, and the Clinton administration began the process leading to the establishment of the National Quality Forum (NQF).

Dr. Robert Wachter, editor of AHRQ *WebM&M*, (the same Dr. Wachter I spoke with in Greenville, SC, in 2010, whom I assume is still keeping me "in mind") held an interview with Janet Corrigan, PhD, then president and CEO of NQF in April 2010. [permission granted]

[As posted on the web site and permission granted]

RW: Tell us what the National Quality Forum does.

JC: The National Quality Forum (NQF) was established in 1999 pursuant to the recommendations of the President's Advisory Commission on Consumer Protection and Quality. Essentially, under the National Technology Transfer and Advancement Act, we are recognized as a private sector standard-setting organization. We review performance measures, best practices, and serious reportable events, and we endorse those as national standards.

RW: Has the fact that you are developing standards fueled public reporting of those standards, or did we need NQF because those initiatives are out there?

JC: Well, it's probably more the former. The fact that we have standardized measures, practices, and serious reportable events, those are tools. They enable reporting efforts. Certainly, there were pioneering public reporting initiatives long before the National Quality Forum came into existence, and there was widespread recognition that we wanted to promote greater transparency back in the 1990s. Fortunately, there was the foresight to establish the National Quality Forum because it's easier if we all agree on standardized measures if they're going to be used in that process.

RW: How well has that agreement gone? You still hear calls for harmonization and that different organizations have their own ways of measuring the same thing.

JC: We've come a long way, actually. The current NQF portfolio includes more than 600 measures, and there will be more coming forward. But volume isn't the issue here. We're trying to get measures that assess important aspects of performance, and measures that are meaningful to consumers. Consumers and purchasers are a very important audience, but measures should also be useful for quality improvement. While we've come a long way in terms of moving toward commonly accepted standardized national measures, we still have challenges when it comes to harmonization. NQF expert panels are asked to identify opportunities to harmonize measures—for example, to make sure that all of the measures in the area of immunizations follow common conventions when it comes to specifying the numerators, the denominators and the exclusions. By harmonizing measure sets, it will make it much easier for current clinicians to understand and use the information to improve patient care.

RW: And what are the carrots and sticks to get everybody to play together?

JC: Well, probably the biggest carrot is when the federal government uses standardized performance measures in its public reporting and payment programs. NQF-endorsed measures are the measures of first choice by the federal government and private purchasers. Medicare, of course, is a very large purchaser, a very large regulator. So they, in many ways, set the stage for standardization and public reporting.

RW: Is the organization agnostic about what happens to the measures? Obviously, you're very well aware of the context and whether measures are being used in no-pay-for-errors or pay- for-performance initiatives. Once a measure is developed and endorsed by the organization, is the organization's role in that measure essentially done?

JC: Well, I wouldn't say it's entirely done. Our primary purpose is to endorse measures that are useful for public reporting and quality improvement purposes. While we don't attempt to pass judgment on specific applications, we encourage everyone to use those tools wisely, given that no measures are perfect. They all have strengths and weaknesses. Our role does continue, though, once a measure goes out the door. We are now working on a more formal feedback loop from the front lines, because we want to know whether measures are performing as expected.

As a part of being endorsed, we do require that the measures be field-tested. But we also realize that the whole area of measurement and public reporting is moving at a very rapid pace, and it is important to have mechanisms for ongoing monitoring. We do review all measures at a minimum every three years, as a part of our maintenance process.

RW: I imagine that the never-ending process of coming up with new measures, while dealing with an ever-increasing set of existing measures that you need to re-review for unintended consequences and new science, must be daunting.

JC: Well, it is, and the other thing is that it's not only daunting, but has made us realize that the whole area of measurement and public reporting needs more focus. That brings me to another major area of responsibility in the National Quality Forum. About three years ago, our Board of Directors expanded the mission of NQF. As I indicated, we were initially established to serve as a private-sector standard-setting organization. And the board looked at the NQF portfolio (which at that time numbered about 150 measures or so, and we now have more than four times that amount), and they realized that the number of measures was increasing rapidly. At the same time, there are gaps in the portfolio. For example, a lot of measures relate to the medical care process, but very few measures address care coordination or handoffs. We don't have as many outcome measures as we would like to assess the impact of healthcare on patient functioning and very few measures of patient engagement in decision-making. So we have a wealth of measures but at the same time, we also have many gaps in the portfolio. The board expanded our mission to include working in partnership with other groups to set national priorities and goals for performance improvement. That effort is now very much under way.

What we have essentially done with those priorities and goals is to identify "high leverage" areas—by which we mean that if we focus our improvement activities on those areas, we will achieve very sizable gains in terms of improved health and healthcare. The *To Err Is Human* and *Crossing the Quality Chasm* reports, I think, set out a direction, a mandate, and a call for very real change. But in all honesty, we haven't seen large improvements in quality or safety, and we haven't really achieved fundamental reform in the delivery system. The delivery system is still fragmented and decentralized. We lack critical supports like electronic health records and personnel health records. By setting national priorities and goals we are also trying to set performance expectations at such a level that meeting these expectations will require more fundamental reform of the delivery system.

RW: You've use the term "shared accountability." What does that mean to you?

JC: We have numerous areas of performance that no individual clinician or even an individual hospital can control. Care coordination is certainly the best example. Medication reconciliation is another good example, as is palliative care. These are all areas were multiple providers—physicians, nurses, pharmacists, health educators, others—contribute to patient outcomes, and the family caregivers are members of the care team as well. In the community, the patient may receive rehabilitative care or home healthcare. All of those providers and healthcare professionals contribute to the patient outcomes. That's an example where we need shared accountability.

Shared accountability is a term that came from some of the work of the Institute of Medicine, where I spent many years. We tried to think through how to encourage all the providers—that touch that patient, that influence the outcomes—to come together and do work to have smooth handoffs, to have good communication, to work within the shared treatment plan to achieve the best outcomes. That's where shared accountability comes in. It's often used in the context of pay-for-performance programs. And right now, we primarily have pay-for-performance programs that reward individual physicians or small practices or perhaps a hospital or a healthcare institution. In the future, we need to move toward shared rewards that reflect that multiple participants need to be held accountable and need to be rewarded for contributing to that patient's outcome.

RW: You mentioned that one of your agendas is to create such a robust and diverse set of measures that systems have to fundamentally reform themselves to meet the mandate. It strikes me that there must be some balance there of just the right number of measures to catalyze change without overwhelming organizations.

JC: Yes. There is a critical balance. And that's the reason that the National Priorities Partnership Effort is underway. Because we realize that right now we probably are overwhelming the front-line delivery system and that we're probably not focusing their efforts on some of the most critical areas. The National Priorities Partnership has identified priorities and goals in six areas—population health, safety, care coordination, palliative and end-of-life care, patient and family engagement, and overuse. Eliminating health disparities is a cross-cutting goal that should be addressed in each of the six priority areas.

The goals in most of these areas are stretch goals—ones that are challenging to achieve, but have great potential to save lives, improve patient outcomes, and remove waste from the healthcare system. We think it's critical to limit that number so that adequate attention can be focused not only on measurement and reporting, but also on the most important thing, which is improvement. Our purchasers and regulators and board certification and recertification groups and accreditors all play critical roles. If they can align their activities around these six areas, we think we have a much better chance of achieving these very significant and difficult goals.

RW: You have a unique perspective on all of this having been at and helped lead the IOM reports on safety and quality. Now we're coming up on the decade anniversary of both reports. What were you expecting to accomplish and what's work the way you thought it would? What's been different?

JC: Well, I'm really pleased about the impact of those two reports. To Err Is Human—in many ways the greatest contribution was that it put safety and quality on the national agenda. When the report came out, it had three days of saturation—level coverage in print and broadcast media. So for the first time safety did become, I think, an issue that the American public became aware of. Not the entire American public, obviously, but a sizable portion of it and the media. And that is very, very important. I believe if you're going to achieve major change in a sector as big and complicated as healthcare, there has to be awareness on the part of the American public and those who represent the American public, i.e., the elected officials, that everything is not okay. So I'm pleased that *To Err Is Human* raised the red flag and said we have to do something here.

RW: Did that response surprise you?

JC: When it was released, we expected quite a bit of media coverage, but not anywhere to the degree that it received. Yes, it was a surprise. Although *To Err Is Human* certainly made a big "splash," *Crossing the Quality Chasm* made important contributions as well. It was one of the very first reports that tied the issue of payment to quality. For the first time, there was awareness that our payment policies have to be modified, even more than they have been already, to be much better aligned with achieving our quality and safety objectives. Now it's taken quite a few years and, frankly, the progress there has been too slow. I hope that we'll engage over the next couple of years in very serious discussions around more fundamental payment reform. What we're doing now with pay-for-performance does begin to tweak the payment mechanisms. But it doesn't go far enough. We're always hearing from the front lines that there are disincentives in our current payment programs that make it difficult to coordinate care for chronically ill patients and to provide the best care, achieve the best outcomes, do it safely, and do it affordable. I hope that we will see more action going forward around payment reform.

Another contribution of *Crossing the Quality Chasm* was a very important chapter about the need for stronger organizational support to achieve higher levels of quality. It called for fundamental reform of the delivery system. That chapter probably received the least attention and I think it's an important one. It's not all about health information technology. That would be a big step forward, and it's critically important that we get electronic health records and personal health records in place and that there be connectivity. But it's also important to recognize that healthcare is so complicated that it's difficult to do it without good knowledge management, without the ability to assemble multidisciplinary teams, without specialized expertise in quality measurement, engineering, and other areas to carefully redesigned care processes. All of that requires more sophisticated organizational supports. That's where we've made the least progress in the last ten years.

~

I included this full interview because I believe Dr. Corrigan clearly presents the efforts of the quality of healthcare army of experts during the past decade or more, and illustrates how my perspective differs on how to reorganize our nation's healthcare delivery system. Perhaps this next, more current, contribution from Dr. Wachter will prove beneficial.

"Is the Patient Safety Movement in Danger of Flickering Out?"
by Dr. Robert Wachter, was posted on his blog on February 18, 2013. [permission granted]

> These should be the best of times for the patient safety movement. After all, it was concerns over medical mistakes that launched the transformation of our delivery and payment models, from one focused on volume to one that rewards performance. The new system (currently a work in progress) promises to put skin in the patient safety game has never before.
>
> Yet I've never been more worried about the safety movement than I am today. My fear is that we will look back on the years between 2000 and 2012 as the "Golden Era of Patient Safety," which would be okay if we'd fixed all the problems. But we have not.
>
> A little history will illuminate my concerns. The modern patient safety movement began with the December 1999 publication of the IOM report on medical errors, which famously documented 44,000–98,000 deaths per year in the US from medical mistakes, the equivalent of a large airplane crash each day. (To illustrate the contrast, we just passed the four-year mark since the last death in a US commercial airline accident.) The IOM report sparked dozens of initiatives designed to improve safety: changes in accreditation standards, new educational requirements, public reporting, promotion of healthcare information technology, and more. It also spawned parallel movements focused on improving quality and patient experience.
>
> As I walk around UCSF Medical Center today, I see an organization transformed by this new focus on improvement. In the patient safety arena, we deeply dissect two to three cases per month using a technique called Root Cause Analysis that I first heard about in 1999. The results of these analyses fuel "system changes"—also a foreign concept to clinicians until recently. We document and deliver care via a state-of-the-art computerized system. Our students and residents learn about QI and safety, and most complete a meaningful improvement project during their training. We no longer receive two years' notice of a Joint Commission accreditation visit; we receive twenty minutes notice. While the national evidence of improvement is mixed, our experience at UCSF reassures me: we've seen lower infection rates, fewer falls, fewer medication errors, fewer

readmissions, better- train clinicians, and better systems. In short, we have an organization that is much better at getting better than it was a decade ago.

So what's the problem? I see two major forces slackening the response to patient safety: clinician (particularly physician) burnout and strategic repositioning by delivery systems to deal with the Affordable Care Act. Like a harried parent rushing out to the car to drive the school carpool, only to discover that he's left his child in the house, we risk leaving behind our precious safety cargo if we fail to ensure that everybody is onboard as we rush headlong into the future.

Let's begin with burnout. When the patient safety field launched in 2000, one might have expected that physicians would be natural foes. After all, say "medical errors" to a practicing doctor and the Pavlovian response is likely to be "malpractice." This reflex made physicians unlikely patient safety enthusiasts, and it is axiomatic that nothing important happens in healthcare if physicians are not engaged.

Yet, by emphasizing systems problems—the "it's not bad people, it's bad systems" argument—many physicians felt validated, some even intrigued and a few (like me) even inspired. Physicians turned from active resisters to, in many cases, real allies.

But the blizzard of new initiatives,—all well meaning but cumulatively overwhelming—thrust at busy clinicians has created overload. The problem, of course, is that nobody freed up the time to do all this new stuff. When commercial airline pilots recertify every year on a simulator, they do this on company time. When they spend thirty minutes completing a preflight checklist, their salary is assured. But for many physicians, these new task—learning a new way of thinking, implementing a checklist, or surviving the installation of a new IT system—are usually obligations on top of an already jam-packed day. Even for nurses, who generally are salaried, new mandates to scan bar codes or even to wash hands ate up precious minutes in days that already lacked much white space.

Although many clinicians have been gratified by their work in safety and quality, I'm afraid this additional work has contributed to high levels of burnout. A recent study in *JAMA Internal Medicine* documented burnout rates significantly higher than those of the rest of the US population—with nearly half of physicians displaying symptoms of burnout. Obviously, patient safety initiatives are not the only cause of this burnout. But the effects on the safety field are very real.

While the statistics are troubling (and, as chair of the ABIM this year, I certainly hear from my share of unhappy doctors), the impact on patient safety really came home during my recent interview of Prof. Bryan Sexton, the Duke sociologists and the world's leading expert on patient safety culture. I had interviewed Bryan about culture six years ago for the federal website I edit, AHRQ *WebM&M*, and I thought it might be a good time to check back in. I approached the interview armed with a bunch of questions, covering things like Executive WalkRounds and teamwork training.

But within ten minutes, I had scrapped all of my questions, because Bryan focused almost entirely on clinician burnout. In his work, he is seeing physicians and nurses so overwhelmed that getting them to think about anything else—safety, quality, teamwork—is nearly impossible. "It's like Maslow's hierarchy," he said, in that people aren't able to focus on higher needs until their basic needs are secured (the full interview will be published in the spring). Because of this, he has shifted his focus to improving "resiliency"—basically, helping docs and nurses restore joy in their work. As Dr. Richard Gunderman points out in a recent article in *The Atlantic*, while reducing dissatisfiers (hassles, bureaucracy, pay cuts, clunky IT systems) is important part of addressing a burnout, "the key (to combating physician burnout) is promoting professional wholeness, which flows from a full understanding of the real sources of fulfillment.

I cling to the hope that improving systems of care will bring fulfillment to clinicians (both from the work itself and the fruits of the labor), as it has for me and many of my colleagues. But it is important to recognize that for many clinicians (and not just the pre-retirement folks), this work is yet one more thing that stands between them and professional satisfaction. The lack of evidence that all our hard work is paying off is also contributing to burnout. Several influential papers using the IHI's Global Trigger Tool methodology, have documented continued high rates of harm; one study of ten hospitals in North Carolina showed no evidence of improvement between 2002 and 2007. On top of that, a steady drumbeat of studies (beautifully chronicled by Brad Flansbaum) demonstrates that nearly every policy intervention that we thought would work (readmission penalties, "no pay for errors," pay for performance, promotion of IT, resident duty-hour reductions) has either failed to work, are has led to negative unanticipated consequences. For people who have given their hearts and souls to making the system work better for patients, the result is more demoralization.

My second major concern about septic patient safety stems from the Affordable Care Act (ACA), one of whose main goals, paradoxically, is to place a premium on value over volume. You'd think that the patient safety field would benefit from such a law (which also includes significant new spending on safety), and perhaps it will . . . eventually. But in the short term, the ACA is yet another speed bump on the road to a safe system.

Just as physicians are overwhelmed and distracted, so too are hospital CEOs and boards. As the healthcare system lurches from its dysfunctional model to a (God willing) better place, healthcare leaders are scrambling to be sure that their organizations have seats when the music stops. The C-suite and boardroom conversations that, a few years ago, were focused on how to make systems better and safer now center on whether to become accountable care organizations, how to achieve alignment with the medical staff, what the insurance exchange will mean for our reimbursement, and the like. To the degree that people remain interested in improving value, here too the emphasis has shifted from the numerator of the value equation (quality, safety, patient experience) to the denominator: cutting cost.

Dr. Gary Kaplan, CEO of Virginia Mason Health System in Seattle, and probably the most admired hospital leader in the country, recently reflected on the state of patient safety in a note to the board of the Lucian Leape Institute at the National Patient Safety Foundation (we're both on the LLI board).

Gary wrote, "(The) reduction in reimbursement and increasing consolidation threatens to make the focus on economics, size, and market competitiveness take precedent over getting better in terms of quality and safety. This will be in part because the 'line of sight' from senior leaders to the front lines of care will be even more distant."

We simply must reorganize our healthcare systems to deliver the highest-value care. Of course, this will require big picture, strategic planning—new relationships, new institutions, new IT systems, and more. It will also depend on the creation of a bottom-up culture that allows those who deliver the care to improve it. Together, this is an awfully full agenda for both leaders and clinicians, and it is a noble one.

But as we proceed, we must remember that healthcare is delivered by real humans, working in organizations that are led by other real humans. Ignoring the pressures that both groups are under may lead us to create lovely systems and dazzling org charts for organizations that continue to harm and kill. In other words, we risk the dystopian world that the great healthcare futurist Ian Morrison has warned of, one in which our hospitals and clinics have the anatomy of high-performing organizations, but not the physiology.

Dr. Wachter asked himself, and others, a profound question: "Is the patient safety movement in danger of flickering out?" But did he answer his own question? If so, how? And how well?

Reread his first two paragraphs. Will the years between 2000 and 2013 become the "Golden Era of Patient Safety" because "they" have fixed all the problems? I think not.

Dr. Wachter sees two major forces slackening the response to patient safety: clinician burnout and strategic repositioning by delivery systems to deal with the Affordable Care Act. I see much lacking in those two "major forces" as the true causes for worry.

Later in his article, Dr. Wachter quotes Dr. Gary Kaplan, CEO of Virginia Mason Health System in Seattle: "(The) reduction in reimbursement and increasing consolidation threatens to make the focus on economics, size, and market competitiveness take precedent over getting better in terms of quality and safety. This will be in part because the 'line of sight' from senior leaders to the front lines of care will be even more distant."

Dr. Wachter closes with, "But as we proceed, we must remember that healthcare is delivered by real humans, working in organizations that are led by other real humans. Ignoring the pressures that both groups are under may lead us to create lovely systems and dazzling org charts for organizations that continue to harm and kill. In other words, we risk the dystopian world that the great healthcare futurist Ian Morrison has warned of, one in which our hospitals and clinics have the anatomy of high-performing organizations, but not the physiology."

Dr. Wachter's soliloquy illustrates the quality of healthcare army of experts' angst, while simultaneously demonstrating their complete failure to recognize every state's obligatory role to create and maintain the organizational structure he alludes to in his last paragraph.

Quality of healthcare army of experts give full meaning to "They can't see the forest for the trees!"

My answer to "Is the patient safety movement in danger of flickering out?": is not only is it "flickering out," it has been "flickering out" since its inception, because those experts fail to recognize the states' responsibility.

There is a fairly simple test to support my conclusion. See if even one of our over forty schools of public health have a department head or professor, who has written, taught, or even spoken on the states' responsibility regarding the healthcare delivery system. "Experts" can't realize the potential importance of a key element they have never recognized. Nowhere in the quality of healthcare army of experts' literature will one find any evidence of their recognition of each state's responsibility. No school of public health wants to take that test.

I regret the need to focus so much attention on one individual, but Dr. Wachter has stepped out in front of so much of the quality of healthcare efforts, I see no other alternative. I do appreciate that his well-publicized offerings provide a clear and distinct difference between our personal philosophies on how to improve the quality of healthcare in America.

The National Quality Forum for Healthcare Measurement and Reporting

The National Quality Forum (NQF) is a nonprofit, nonpartisan, public service organization established by Congress in January 1998 for the purpose of promoting the quality, appropriateness, and effectiveness of healthcare. The NQF process is to arrange for the development, periodic review and updating of:

1. Clinically relevant guidelines that may be used by physicians, educators, and healthcare practitioners to assist in determining how diseases, disorders, and other health conditions can most effectively and appropriately be prevented, diagnosed, treated, and managed clinically.
2. Standards of quality, performance measures, and medical review criteria through which healthcare providers and other appropriate entities may assess or review the provision of healthcare and assure the quality of such care.

The NQF mission is "to improve the quality of American healthcare by building consensus on national priorities and goals for performance improvement and working in partnership to achieve them; endorsing national consensus standards for measurement and public reporting on performance; and promoting the attainment of national goals through education and outreach programs. The NQF vision includes establishing national priorities and goals to achieve healthcare that is safe, timely, beneficial, patient-centered, equitable and efficient.

NQF, in 2002, created and endorsed a list of serious reportable events (SREs) to increase public accountability and consumer access to critical information about healthcare performance. Twenty-seven SREs are classified under one of the six categories: surgical, product or device, patient-protection, care management, environment, or criminal. (The SRE report was revised in 2006 and again beginning in 2011.)

Examples of SRE Surgical Events:
- Surgery performed on the wrong body part.
- Surgery performed on the wrong person.
- Wrong surgical procedure performed on a patient.
- Unintended retention of a foreign object in a patient after surgery or other procedure.
- Intra-operative or immediately postoperative death in an ASA Class I patient (i.e. 27 y.o. female for minor knee surgery under local anesthesia).

The Serious Reportable Events report (sixty pages), now undergoing its second revision, represents considerable time, effort, and cost, involving numerous healthcare experts classifying multiple unintended patient care events that have been occurring within our healthcare delivery system throughout its history. What is not mentioned in that sixty-page report is: Who should those SREs be reported to in any of our nation's hospitals (and surgery centers), and what accountability mechanism might be available for a proper response?

Dr. Kenneth Kizer, NQF first president and CEO (1998–2006) introduced the term *never events* in 2001 in reference to particularly shocking medical errors (such as wrong-site surgery) that should *never* occur. *Surgery Journal* provided the following article in December 2012 coauthored by Doctors Pronovost, Makary, and others, that offers more current *never event* consideration.

Surgical Never Events in the United States, Pronovost, P., Makary, M., et al., *Surgery Journal*, December 2012 [permission not granted, therefore paraphrased]

The authors acknowledged that surgical never events are used as *"quality metrics"*, while at the same time no one has an understanding regarding the cost of these events, the patient outcomes, or the medical capabilities of the doctors involved in these events, therefore their study was an attempt to describe the above using paid malpractice claims associated with such events.

National Practitioner Data Bank was their source for information they deemed necessary for their study. Using slightly less than 10,000 paid malpractice claims for surgical never events between 1990 and 2010 the authors concluded that surgical never events are costly to the healthcare system, are associated with serious harm to patients, and they hoped this study might "help guide prevention strategies".

My Response: Doctors Pronovost, Makary, and their coauthors are to be commended for their effort to bring increased consideration to one of the most serious, negative aspects of our current healthcare delivery system. However, the National Practitioner Data Bank is, and has always been, a highly flawed "federal repository" for those seeking meaningful understanding of the true extent of questionable patient care.

Medical malpractice claims and medical malpractice litigation (Sue or forget it) results have never, and can never, provide a realistic depiction of the subject of their article. I suggest that the culprit in the subject of their article is the state's (every state's) failure to create a far better method of obtaining the urgently needed information these authors appear to be seeking. Those authors and I can certainly agree that the subject of their article is far greater than known, and far more costly than ever estimated in loss of life, loss of quality of life, and, of course, loss of great sums of money.

Janet M. Corrigan, PhD, MBA, (one of the three co-editors of *To Err Is Human*) and interviewee with Dr. Wachter at his *WebM&M* program retired as president and CEO of NQF in mid-2012. The Lucian Leape Institute, at the National Patient Safety Foundation announced, effective July 1, 2012, Dr. Corrigan as the newest member of that Foundation. Dr. Christine K. Cassel was made the new NQF president and CEO as of July 1, 2013.

Institute for Healthcare Improvement, (IHI) Cambridge, Massachusetts, [quoted from the IHI web site, permission granted]

> IHI was founded in the late 1980s by Dr. Don Berwick and a group of visionary individuals committed to redesigning healthcare into a system without errors, waste, delay, and unsustainable costs. Since then, we've grown from an initial collection of grant-supported programs to a self-sustaining organization with worldwide influence.
>
> In our first decade, we focused on the identification and subsequent spread of best practices. This work reduced defects and errors in microsystems such as the emergency department or the intensive care unit.
>
> In our second decade, we established a defining focus on innovation, R&D, and the bold creation of new solutions to old problems. We reinvented multidimensional systems of care and began transforming entire systems. This work manifested in the renown 100,000 Lives Campaign and 5 Million Lives Campaign, spreading best practice changes to thousands of US hospitals in creating a vibrant worldwide improvement community.
>
> As we entered our third decade, we recognized a new need for healthcare as a complete social, geopolitical enterprise. To accelerate the path to the health and care we need, IHI created the triple aim, a framework for optimizing health system performance by simultaneously focusing on the health of a population, the experience of care for individuals within that population, and the per capita cost of providing that care.
>
> Today, IHI is an influential force in health and healthcare improvement in the US and has a rapidly growing footprint and dozens of other nations, including Canada, England, Scotland, Denmark, Sweden, Singapore, Latin America, New Zealand, Ghana, Malawi, and South Africa.

Our Vision and Mission

An Irish proverb says that "When you come upon a wall, throw your hat over it, and then go get your hat." At IHI, the spirit of this one little saying has inspired many big outcomes. People who are drawn to IHI see beyond walls to the possibilities on the other side. We are inspired and energized by one uniting vision: a future in which everyone has the best care and health possible.

Although the problems are big and daunting, we resolve to approach them with optimism grounded in rigorous science, hard work, and a relentless drive for results.

IHI is a recognized and generous leader, a trustworthy partner, in the first place to turn for expertise, help, and encouragement for anyone, anywhere who wants to change healthcare profoundly for the better.

Dr. Don Berwick is the immediate past administrator of the Center for Medicare and Medicaid Services. IHI held its first Annual National Forum in 1988 and its 24th Annual Forum in December 2012.

The IHI Triple Aim
1. To improve the health of the population,
2. To enhance the patient experience of care, and
3. To control the cost of care.

> "I believe the IHI Triple Aim is designed to change the course of healthcare history ... And I believe South Carolina is going to be one of the first states to prove it."
>
> ~Maureen Bisognano, President and CEO of IHI

South Carolina Triple Aim efforts are led by BlueCross Blue Shield of SC, Health Sciences South Carolina, and South Carolina Hospital Association, and supported by several dozen additional agencies, organizations, and alliances. As seen in the next chapter, South Carolina has been chosen to be the initial test site for their concerted efforts by both IHI and Dr. Gawande's Checklist Manifesto and Joint Commission High Reliability.

Because of the enormity of IHI efforts to improve healthcare here and around the world, only one other example of those efforts is offered here.

Respectful Management of Serious Clinical Adverse Events

This white paper introduces an overall approach and tools designed to support two processes: the proactive preparation of a plan for managing serious clinical adverse events, and the reactive emergency response of an organization that has no such plan.

Executive Summary

"You just heard at this morning's CEO leadership meeting that a forty-year-old father of five children died in the surgical ICU last night, hours after receiving medication intended for another patient. Everyone is upset. Questions are flying around the hospital: What does the family know? Who did it? What happened? What can we say? Would the patient have died anyway? (He was very sick). Has anyone gone to the press?

Every day, clinical adverse events occur within our healthcare system, causing physical and psychological harm to one or more patients, their families, staff (including medical staff), the community, and the organization. In the crisis that often emerges, what differentiates organizations, positively or negatively, is there culture of safety; the role of the board of trustees and executive leadership; advanced planning for such an event; the balance prioritization of the needs of the patient and family, staff, and organization; hand how actions immediately and over time address the integrated elements of empathy, disclosure, support (including reimbursement), assessment, resolution (including compensation), learning, and improvement. The risks of not responding to these adverse events in a timely and effective manner are significant, and include loss of trust, absence of healing, no learning and improvement, the sending of mixed messages about what is really important to the organization, increased likelihood of regulatory action or lawsuits, and challenges by the media.

From time to time, IHI receives urgent requests from organizations seeking help in the aftermath of a serious clinical adverse event, including: What should we do? Who should do it? What should we say, and to whom? Among the most striking attributes of these requests is that, most often, the organization is building its response from the ground up, not from an existing clinical crisis management plan. In responding to such requests, IHI draws on the fields of patient- and family-centered care, patient safety, service recovery, crisis management, and disaster planning—as well as the learning assembled from many courageous organizations over the last fifteen years that have tried to manage these crises, initially and over time, respectfully and effectively. IHI also has met many patients, family members, and healthcare staff (the so-called "second victims"), many of whom are rightfully angry and frustrated over the disrespectful treatment they received after clinical adverse events.

The development of this white paper was motivated by three objectives:
- Encourage and help every organization to develop a clinical crisis management plan before they need to use it;
- Provide an approach to integrating this plan into the organizational culture of quality and safety, with a particular focus on patient-and family-centered care and fair and just treatment for staff; and
- Provide organizations with a concise, practical resource to inform their efforts when a serious adverse event occurs in the absence of a clinical crisis management plan and/or culture of quality and safety.

In furtherance of these objectives, this paper includes three tools for leaders—a Checklist, a Work Plan, and an Assessment Tool—and numerous resources to guide practice (See Appendix).

Definition of a Serious Clinical Adverse Event

In any healthcare clinical setting, adverse events occur frequently. This white paper focuses particularly on those clinical adverse events with an impact of permanent psychological and/ or physical harm (or death) on one patient are many, often referred to as sentinel events. These are events that are included in categories G, H, and I in the National Coordinating Council for Medication Error Reporting and Prevention (NCC MERP) harm index. The National Quality Forum Serious Reportable Events provides another baseline list of serious clinical events. Healthcare Performance Improvements (HPI) has developed the Safety Event Classification and the Serious Safety Event Rate, with common definitions and an algorithm for the classification of safety events based on the degree of harm. For the purposes of this white paper, the type of harm on which we focus is usually, but not exclusively, preventable. Of note, many of the most challenging and poorly handled serious clinical adverse events occur when too much time is spent on determining preventability and not enough on empathy and support.

Obviously, great effort, by many highly educated and dedicated experts has gone into the development of a plan whereby hospital administrators, boards of trustees, medical and nursing staffs, and all others involved can respond in a well-organized manner when one of the estimated 200,000 needless hospital *never events* occurs (plus non-fatal adverse events and events within surgery centers, etc.). Where are the states and their responsibility to "regulate," plus the century-old state medical examining boards? As one learns more, each person is left with a personal decision

Patient-Centered Outcomes Research Institute (PCORI)

Snapshots of just a few of the components of the quality of healthcare army of experts will conclude with a brief look at the "new kid" on the quality of healthcare block, created by Congress in 2010.

About Us [quoted from web site with permission]
The Patient Centered Outcomes Research Institute (PCORI) is authorized by Congress to conduct research to provide information about the best available evidence to help patients and their healthcare providers make more informed decisions. PCORI's research is intended to give patients a better understanding of the prevention, treatment and care options available, and the science that supports those options.

Mission

The Patient-Centered Outcomes Research Institute (PCORI) helps people make informed healthcare decisions, and important healthcare delivery and outcomes, by producing and promoting high integrity, evidence-based information that comes from research guided by patients, caregivers and the broader healthcare community.

Vision

Patients and the public have the information they need to make decisions that reflect their desired health outcomes.

Patient-Centered Outcomes Research (PCORI) helps people and their caregivers communicate and make informed healthcare decisions, allowing their voices to be heard in assessing the value of healthcare options. This research answers patient-centered questions such as:

1. "Given my personal characteristics, conditions and preferences, what should I expect will happen to me?"
2. "What are my options and what are the potential benefits and harms of those options?"
3. "What can I do to improve the outcomes that are most important to me?"
4. "How can clinicians and the care delivery systems they work in help me make the best decisions about my health and healthcare?"

To answer those questions, PCORI:
- Assesses the benefits and harms of preventive, diagnostic, therapeutic, palliative, or health delivery system interventions to inform decision making, highlighting comparisons and outcomes that matter to people;
- Is inclusive of an individual's preferences, autonomy and needs, focusing on outcomes that people notice and care about such as survival, function, symptoms, and health related quality of life;
- Incorporates a wide variety of settings and diversity of participants to address individual differences and barriers to implementation and dissemination; and
- Investigates (or may investigate) optimizing outcomes while addressing burden to individuals, availability of services, technology, and personnel, and other stakeholder perspectives.

South Carolina Business Coalition on Health

Annual Meeting May 8, 2012, Greenville, South Carolina

The first half of this all-day meeting consisted of four outstanding presentations by speakers illustrating successful methods that have been used in various parts of the nation helping healthcare systems better control the rising cost of healthcare.

The afternoon consisted of two sessions, each with three different workshops that the attendees could choose from. I attended the two sessions focused on South Carolina's collaboration with IHI in their Triple Aim endeavor.

While one could only be impressed with the very positive efforts across the nation to confront the cost and access aspects of our huge healthcare dilemma, I was also struck by the absence of any recognition of the quality of healthcare issues, and in particular, the growing needless hospital death tragedy. Within two days after attending that meeting, I had composed several thought papers, one centered on patient centeredness.

Patient Centeredness: 3 Counterpoints

IOM: Patient centeredness is healthcare that establishes a partnership among practitioners, patients, and their families to ensure that decisions respect patients "wants, needs, and preferences" and that patients have the education and support they need to make decisions and participate in their own care. Patient centeredness "encompasses qualities of compassion, empathy, and responsiveness to the needs, values, and expressed preferences of the individual patient.

Speaking against patient centeredness is like speaking against motherhood, the flag, and apple pie, but I still wish to offer these thoughts for discussion.

1. Arrogant and egotistical doctors excepted, most doctors (yours truly included), think and feel as though we are (*were* in my case) trying to do that with all of our patients. If half the audience was doctors, what do you think they would be thinking about patient centeredness?
2. Some estimate that 50 percent or more of all healthcare problems in our nation are self-induced by unhealthy lifestyles. (List them). So, doctors are to fulfill all of the above prerequisites for patient centeredness for all of those patients who are their own worst enemies?
3. Needless hospital deaths—twenty-plus years ago—98,000 (268 a day). Current estimated rate approaches double. What should be priority number one regarding the quality of healthcare in America? A long track record of needless hospital deaths and a twelve-year IOM record of promise to reduce by 50 percent in five years should deserve far more consideration.

Patient centeredness is a positive concern regarding patient care that should be considered within the full context of the doctor/patient relationship, but questionable patient care accountability should take precedent in the current national effort to improve the quality of healthcare in America.

What patient centeredness activists fail to understand is that my efforts to greatly increase the fair and meaningful use of medical peer review and greatly diminish the use of "Sue or forget it" (medical malpractice litigation) will provide far more true patient centeredness than their current mantra.

Example: More than three decades ago, I created a full-page informed consent for my major surgery patients. I strongly urged adults to bring another person with them for their initial consultation, and I gave them a copy of that informed consent form with this instruction: "Talk about what I have told you during the consultation during your trip home, read the informed consent, and write any questions you might have on the back. IF you decide to have the surgery, don't sign the informed consent until I have answered all of your questions satisfactorily." I still have copies of my informed consent forms.

Patient care accountability *must begin* with a functional system of medical peer review in every hospital in America that is reasonably fair to both doctor and patient. I know how to create such a system, and I have said so in two previous books. Patient Centered Outcomes Research Institute efforts might give my offer consideration.

An article appeared in the *Patient Safety & Quality Healthcare Journal* in 2007:

"We're Not Your Enemy: An Appeal From a Consumer to Re-imagine to Tort Reform"
by Susan S. Sheridan, MIM, MBA, and Martin J. Hatlie, JD.

The major thrust of the article is a plea to make tort reform caps more equitable for those injured by negligent care, or their surviving kin. Ms. Sheridan's introduction to safety issues—and her motivation to make a difference—came through grave medical errors, which led to longstanding needs for her son, and the loss of her husband.

While I join them in seeking the same goal, greater patient safety, I believe the best route to take in order to reach that goal is to replace "Sue or forget it" (medical malpractice litigation) with meaningful medical peer review, because tort reform is only the caboose of that litigation process.

My initial interest in this article steams from its title, "We're Not Your Enemy," which raises several questions for me:

Who is the enemy in the quest to make healthcare safer? Who determines who the "enemy" is?

What qualifies those to make such judgments?

Why is anyone considered the enemy when the need is so great? Both authors are on the advisory board of the *Patient Safety & Quality Healthcare Journal,* and both deserve further recognition.

Sue Sheridan was named PCORI Director of Patient Engagement in 2012, and has led the World Health Organization's Patients for Patient Safety initiative.

Martin Hatlie was the coauthor of the AMA chapter-long contribution to the 1989 book, *Medical Malpractice Solutions.* That article, "The Model Medical Liability and Patient Protection Act: A Fault-Based Administrative System for Resolving Medical Malpractice Claims," outlined the AMA quest for special medical malpractice courts that began in 1988 and quietly disappeared in the mid-1990s.

Mr. Hatlie then became the AMA founding director of the National Patient Safety Foundation in 1997, at the same time that the AMA House of Delegates was taking their first of four annual votes making expert witness testimony equal to patient care, and ultimately leading to the creation of the Litigation Center of the AMA that will be described in detail in Chapter 5.

This next point will really get me in trouble.

The press release headline said, "Governor Nikki Haley, DHEC, DSS, & DHHS to announce collaborative effort to improve health"

> COLUMBIA, SC—Governor Nikki Haley, Catherine Templeton, director of the South Carolina Department of Health and Environmental Control (DHEC), Lillian Koller, director of the South Carolina Department of Social Services (DSS), Dr. Marion Burton, medical director of the South Carolina Department of Health and Human Services (DHHS), and Dr. Janice Keys, director of the Medical University of South Carolina's Boeing Center for Children's Wellness, on Thursday will announce plans to work together with medical and nutritional experts, farmers, grocers, private employers, and Supplemental Nutrition Assistance Program (SNAP) participants to fight obesity and improve health in South Carolina.
>
> The announcement is scheduled for Thursday, February 21, 2013 at 1:30 p.m. at DHEC as part of the agency's quarterly "Unified! A Voice Against Obesity" statewide meeting.
>
> WHO: Gov. Nikki Haley, DHEC Director Catherine Templeton, DSS Director Lillian Koller, DHHS's Dr. Marion Burton, and MUSC's Dr. Janice Keys
>
> WHAT: Announcement regarding South Carolina's fight against obesity and to improve health
>
> WHEN: Thursday, February 21, 1:30 p.m.

Like speaking against patient centeredness, no one in their right mind could be against a concerted effort to confront our crippling healthcare issues due to obesity, resulting in our growing diabetes and adult onset type 2 diabetes catastrophe, right?

I am not against their effort – I just don't see how they can ever hope to be even marginally successful. They are really talking about individual behavior modification on a massive scale. A very large percent of their state's entire population can qualify for inclusion in their great endeavor. But don't take my word for how difficult this problem is. Parade Magazine published an article in March 2013 by Dr. Howard McMahan called "A Day in the Life of a Country Doctor."

Dr. McMahan has spent over twenty years in Ocilla, Georgia (population 3,414), three hours south of Atlanta, as the only doctor within miles. He knows all his patients by name—and often their parents and grandparents as well, and he has a growing number of patients who are battling chronic diseases like diabetes and emphysema. Yet he finds it very difficult, and usually impossible to get those who desperately need to, to change their lifestyle, i.e., improved diet, exercise, you know the drill.

If people who know and love their doctor, who knows them by their names, won't change their harmful lifestyles for him, how are Governor Haley, state healthcare agencies, medical and nutritional experts, farmers, grocers, private powers, and the army of quality of healthcare experts going to achieve success?

The problem is that the "system" is broken! Or more precisely, the "system" is a non-system. So they are trying to incrementally change a system none of them can describe, and in fact, no one has ever even attempted to describe. I actually know how to do that—but the governor, et al., first feel the need to make most people in South Carolina thinner and healthier.

I am NOT against that. But I will only believe it when (if) I see it.

These efforts will not work due to flaws in our current healthcare delivery system:

- It is unorganized and dysfunctional (a non-system).
- It is devoid of accountability.
- It is becoming more and more problematic, in spite of great effort by a multitude of "healthcare experts."
- Abraham Flexner confronted similar problems in medical education in both America and Canada. In 1910 his *Flexner Report* "began the process" leading to solving that great problem by first determining: "Where are we now, and how did we get here?" He next duplicated his process in Western Europe with similar success. We have several role models, like his, for what needs to be done—but those models are ignored.

Healthcare Role Models

1. Abraham Flexner—Where are we now, and how did we get here?
2. Defense Department—Organizational structure with clearly defined points of authority, delegated authority, responsibility, and accountability.
3. The US space program to put men on the moon—various segments of expertise come under a big tent with one goal.

Einstein—who pointed out that continuing to do things the same way while seeking a different result is the definition of insanity.

Machiavelli said to change an existing system would be *almost impossible*, but that doesn't mean it can't be done, or that someone shouldn't try.

This is only the beginning. For those who want a better understanding of their healthcare delivery system, its many problems, and the army of quality of healthcare experts' efforts to make it better, there is far more. As that old song goes, *"We've only just begun,"* or rather, I have only just begun.

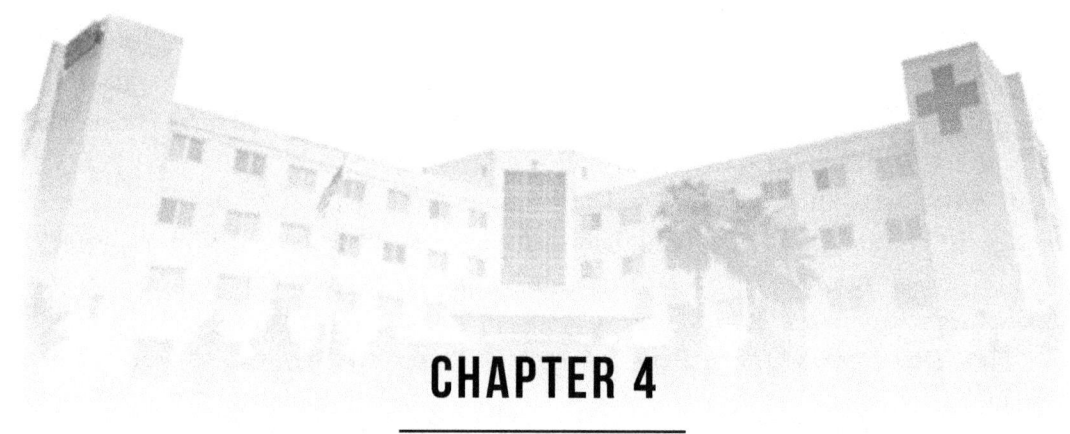

CHAPTER 4

QUALITY OF HEALTHCARE IMPROVEMENT EFFORTS

Compare and Contrast

To reiterate what I said in my email to Dr. Wachter in 2010: "I am as passionate as anyone you know in wanting to contribute to making healthcare better." However, I do not believe any person, myself included, has a right to speak publicly about healthcare improvement matters and not be willing to have what they offer be questioned.

The past twenty-plus year quality of healthcare track record is what it is, and that dismal track record demands to be questioned in an open and transparent manner. Therefore I will compare and contrast two wonderful examples of efforts to improve the quality of healthcare in our nation's hospitals. The first example is supplied by the same Dr. Wachter. I have included in its entirety the transcript of a ten-minute audio excerpt taken from the interview between Mr. Boothman and Dr. Wachter supplied by the AHRQ *WebM&M*: Perspective Print View. [permission granted]

AHRQ WebM&M, morbidity and mortality rounds on web. "In Conversation with Richard C. Boothman, JD," March 2012 [with permission]

> *Editor's note:* Rick Boothman, an attorney, is the chief risk officer for the University of Michigan Health System. After many years as a trial lawyer, Mr. Boothman joined the University in 2001, and soon developed a pioneering approach to medical mistakes and risk management, one emphasizing an honest approach to errors, early apology, and rapid settlement offers when the system was at fault. This approach, which has been demonstrated to lower malpractice payouts, has been emulated widely.

Interview

Dr. Robert Wachter, editor, AHRQ *WebM&M*: Tell us a little bit about your background.

Richard C. Boothman: All through my career as a trial lawyer, I wondered to myself what a tough way it is to resolve disputes. Interestingly, in my first trial I was representing a surgeon, and at the end of the two-week trial, as the jury was filing out of the box and the lady who sued leaned around the podium and said to the surgeon, "If I had known everything that I heard in this courtroom I would never have sued you in the first place," I remember thinking that there's got to be a better way to handle this. That was the first time in six years she had spoken to a physician with whom she had a very intimate relationship before things went bad. So I suppose the seeds of what later became my career choices were planted early on.

RW: When you had that epiphany after that case with the surgeon—that there needed to be a different approach to disclosure—what was your view of what needed to be different in the system?

RB: It developed gradually, but relatively early on as a trial lawyer I started a practice of sending a letter back to my clients that I called a "litigation discharge summary." The letter would summarize the issues in the case and the course of the case, but then include recommendations at the end. Things like, you might think about x, y, and z, which might have avoided this lawsuit. What I found was a startling silence at the other end and even some resistance, where clients would literally tell me, "We hired you to handle the malpractice case. Thank you very much, but we didn't ask for any opinions about how we could change our clinical care, or whether we should have pursued peer review for this challenged doctor." I was startled by the psychological separation.

I've since come to realize that we may have made a Faustian bargain many years ago when medicine first started turfing these complex issues to a profession that is trained to fight. As a lawyer, I'm not trained to know right or wrong. I'm really trained to win the case, and the concept behind the American judicial system is that, with vigorous advocates on both sides, usually the truth will win out. When you think back to the idea of turfing these issues to lawyers before we even understand them, we got exactly what we bargained for—an adversarial system. Somewhere along the way it occurred to me that the open access to the courtroom is in some ways the crown jewel of our democracy, but we've perverted the purposes and created this as a first resort rather than the last resort it's intended to be. It's a decidedly expensive and risky way to resolve disputes that should be resolved, or attempted to be resolved, through other means.

RW: Why do you think the system evolved that way?

RB: It's complex, but to boil it down I believe that we're all hardwired to avoid confrontation. That's part of the fight or flight response. With healthcare providers of all stripes, you have a self-selected group that really doesn't like that kind of confrontation. It was handy and it was comfortable to be able to rid themselves of having to deal with that, at least in the acute phase. To be able to hold your hand up and say to somebody who's angry with you, "This is what I have insurance for, go talk to my lawyer." There are also some economic drivers to shift the financial risk and exposure of financial consequences to an insurance company rendered this a business decision and a piece of business overhead. Instead of worrying about the enormous verdict, they could just look at their insurance premium as a line item on their balance sheet and it became predictable. In the early days of my career, you didn't see very many catastrophic verdicts in medical malpractice. That's a relatively recent occurrence when you think back to the decades of malpractice litigation. It may have made sense to shift the financial risk and the insurance model back in the 1970s, but today the consequence of doing that has been significant. It divorced the accountability for the bad results from the clinicians who are really best situated to fix the problems that gave rise to the unanticipated outcome, and it foisted it to a profession that is built for fighting. We got just what we asked for, an adversarial process.

RW: So when you came to Michigan and proposed the way the system should work and it's fundamentally different—almost turned on its head—from the system that you're inheriting. How did people receive that?

RB: Well, I built on a lot of things that people before me had in place. I'd like to think what I accomplished was really a form of permission. It was not a hard sell. In the first month I was here, I was able to distill down to three simple principles, at least as far as its claims were concerned, what the university should be about. Oddly enough they were seen at the time as revolutionary, but I don't know anybody who can argue with them. They're very simply, if we hurt somebody through inappropriate medical care, it is the ethic and culture of this place to do our best to quickly make it right in a reasonable way—to apologize and compensate fairly and quickly. The second principle was actually more foreign to this place, and that was that we ask much of caregivers who work in an inherently risky environment with inherently risky modalities. They can't control all of the risk. In other words, caregivers can do all the right and reasonable things and still end up with unanticipated outcomes. We owe them support too. The situation I inherited when I came to the University of Michigan was that we were risk averse enough that we were even settling cases where we felt we did not make a mistake. So that second principle had to be that, where our care was deemed reasonable, where we did not adversely impact the outcome, our caregivers deserved our full support. The third principle, which was the most radical at the time, was by all means we should learn from our patients' experiences, we should learn from our mistakes, and infuse in our system those lessons learned as quickly as possible.

Not wait the two to five years litigation can take to run its course and then put all the other interval patients at risk.

Those are the three simple principles: to compensate when we've acted badly, to support our staff when we've acted reasonably, and to learn from our experiences. Once I distilled those down to the three simple principles, it created constancy about how we were responding to these events. We weren't just reacting to some cases that posed big financial risks and other cases that didn't. We shifted it from a game mentality—that is, we were no longer asking ourselves, "Can we win in court?" We were asking ourselves, "Did we make a mistake?" "Did we act reasonably under the circumstances?" That in itself was a big shift from litigation gamesmanship to a more fundamental question that I knew we could answer for ourselves. We didn't need a court to answer, "Was our care reasonable, and did it meet our standards under the circumstances?" Once you start taking control and feel that you're in control over that question, it actually brings a sense of calm and personal accountability, or institutional accountability, over these difficult situations. But even so we started small: one case at a time. I publicized the good results, both ways, the settlements that happened early and spared our doctors litigation, also cases where the patients finally were convinced that we didn't do anything wrong and we avoided a lawsuit that might have happened earlier.

RW: Was your theory in moving in this direction that not only was this the right thing to do but there would ultimately be economic advantages in it? Obviously the data has supported that notion, but I think for many people that was a big surprise.

RB: Actually, the cost savings were never a doubt in my mind. In fact, years later people were irritated with me because I did not compulsively keep metrics as is the habit in an academic institution. My feeling was that this was just common sense. I had no doubt that, even in the cases we had to settle by stepping up early and settling, I'd get a more favorable settlement and we would avoid the transactional costs. The counter-intuitive part was keyed to that second principle. It's quite common in litigation circles to see cases that are strong defense cases as cases we should still settle to avoid the attorney fees. Early on when we tried cases sometimes at a cost that was as much as three times what it would have cost to settle the case, that was a challenge to make that argument. That we have a large audience out there of plaintiff's lawyers and patients and consumers and even judges, and they need to see that we are acting in a principled way, even if it doesn't seem to make sense from a cost-effective perspective on that case. One of the early cases we tried was a case that ultimately I could have settled for $40,000 or fifty thousand dollars and it cost me three times that to try it. But, it was very important for us to make that point, not only to the plaintiff's bar that was watching, but also to our own staff that we would stand firm and not just succumb to the early easy business practice of expedient settlements.

RW: How do you figure out which bucket cases fall in?

RB: The vast majority of cases are shades of gray, very few are black and white, and that's been an interesting evolution. When we first started we often would ask ourselves, "Can we find experts to support the care that we rendered in the given case?" We quickly morphed into a more personal question, "Is this the care that we expected of ourselves under those circumstances?" And to understand that requires you to really understand the circumstances. Simply put, I want doctors to always wash their hands before they touch me, but if I come into the emergency room with a stab wound to my neck please don't stop at the sink, just get your hand over that bleeding. The circumstances matter and we had to work hard to figure that out. That was second nature to me as a trial lawyer with twenty years of experience. So I guess the short answer is that yes, they all have shades of gray, but it is in the nature of academic medicine to know what is expected and what is not expected under the circumstances.

It really isn't as hard as you might think to answer whether this is the care that we expect of ourselves or not. Do we always get it right? No, I've defended some cases that we probably shouldn't have defended and realized during litigation that we should settle. Have we settled cases that maybe we didn't need to? Yes, that's probably true too. But overall, it's quite dramatic when you look at the difference in our experience. Our director of risk management, Susan Anderson, created a graph that was very eye opening, even for me. Looking at cases that we settled over the last ten or fifteen years, we compared them by the number of cases that we have concluded our care was reasonable versus not; before 2001, more than 50 percent of the settlements were in cases that we believed we did not violate the standard of practice and yet we still settled those cases. There has been a complete flip since then. Today it's rare that we pay on a case we have concluded we did not violate the standard of practice.

What that translates to in my mind is two things. One is we have taken control over the quality of this dialogue for ourselves. We've said to the system, this isn't first about malpractice. This is about our own accountability, and we will stand firm both ways. That's important. We've also weeded out almost all of the cases that were brought formerly where we still thought our care was reasonable. We don't see those cases anymore because we've proactively talked to the patient, changed the nature of the quality of that dialogue, and we're avoiding the cases that might have been brought in the past.

Where we find ourselves is kind of interesting. When I started at any given time we had roughly 250 to 300 lawsuits, it would vacillate. Today we're down to eighty to ninety, but we haven't broken below eighty, and that's troubling to me. What we find is that in the majority of those cases, we believe we are at fault. So the next frontier is to start to take a hard look at those because we don't have excuses anymore. We can't blame the plaintiff's bar and we can't blame opportunistic patients. We ourselves have concluded that the residual cases, after we've pared away those groundless lawsuits, are really ours to deal with, and I think the single biggest benefit to a transparent and honest approach is that we've finally gotten rid of all of those excuses.

RW: How do you think about risk management and patient safety in terms of how they've acted with each other traditionally and what you're trying to do now?

RB: Well, it's actually fascinating and I am more invigorated than ever over this. Right now, we are asking this question: "What is it about the remaining eighty to ninety cases that we could have intervened in had we only asked the right questions or had we only paid attention to the right information?" We are now convinced that we're not sampling those pockets of information that every health system has but doesn't tap. A simple example is a comment that one of our surgeons made to me about two weeks ago. He said to me, "I was on faculty here six months, at only six months I could give you a short list of people I never wanted to be in an operating room with." That information is well known. We just need to make greater efforts to tap it and then act on it. Who are those people that everybody knows about who may be unsafe or may be challenged? Maybe we need to get our arms around them and make them safer. I think that's the next frontier. So what we've managed to do is eliminate the noise. If you think of it as a researcher might, we've eliminated all the variables, but we're down to the cases that are our responsibility. I'm confident we could cut this number yet again by a third, or even a half, just by asking questions that historically we've never asked.

RW: It's interesting when you talk about what the surgeon told you, it was not about, "Here's a system that's dysfunctional and needs to be fixed." It got more into the notion of individual quality or personal relationships, which is a harder nut to crack. So that surgeon says to you, "Here are people who everybody knows are unsafe." Play that forward, now you know that, what do you do?

RB: First of all, interestingly, getting the names is hard. In that conversation I slid a legal pad across the table and I said, "Write them down and I'll start looking at them," and he wouldn't write them down. There's a complex question about what to do next. First with the culture change: peer review, for instance, has traditionally meant that we wait until somebody bottoms out, until someone has become such an embarrassment or so utterly unsafe that we can't ignore it anymore, then we pluck them out and engage in a very messy and risky process of pulling their privileges or submitting them to a licensing board. That's our shame. We need to get out in front of these people before they become an embarrassment and before they hurt a lot of people. So we're doing a number of things here that are very exciting.

Dr. Skip Campbell [the chief medical officer] has revolutionized peer review. He's made it relevant. He's made it embracing, not disciplinary. We are going to great lengths to identify those outliers based on provable metrics that are relevant to the specialty involved. Instead of seeing people as ultimately disposable, we're getting our arms around them and we're enrolling them in various programs to help them with communication skills or understand why they're challenged. The next frontier is various ways to take advantage of collections of information that we haven't historically tapped. So why not sample the residents quarterly in an anonymous way and just ask them, "What's on your mind? What are you worried about? Who are you worried about?" People won't report if they believe it will always be disciplinary. So we have to move this culture in tandem. We have to convince people that we care about them. We understand that sometimes good people can go astray a little bit, and we can get on top of those things and make them safer—not just dispose of them when they become an embarrassment. So sampling patients, sampling residents, sampling the nursing staff—you go to a floor and just ask, "What keeps you up at night?"

The one thing I would twist a little bit is that I think the notion that was very popular a few years ago—that we should not look at personal accountability but instead create a blameless culture—was misguided. Even beneath processes that are challenged are responsible individuals. If we change the feel of it from punitive to progressive, we won't feel so badly and we won't work so hard to avoid personal accountability. When there's a challenged individual, it's not just the individual who may have a problem, it may be the manager, division chief, or department chair who was well aware of that problem but did nothing. We need to understand these deeper root causes that just put a bandage over the visible problem. We're even revolutionizing our root cause analysis process here because it did not historically really get to the root causes. When a surgeon thinks that it's acceptable to do two surgeries at one time (notwithstanding the increased infection risk, the distraction, putting residents in situations that they're not well qualified for, or putting patients at risk), the root cause of that is probably a financial one. Maybe an eat-what-you-kill compensation system puts perverse incentives in front of people and causes them to take risks that they shouldn't be taking. We need to be robust enough to start asking those harder questions if we're going to make a difference in this last frontier.

RW: You're talking about tackling a lot of hot button issues: peer review, economic incentives that drive behavior, recasting the balance between no blame and accountability. How does the brand new risk manager at a 150-bed community hospital in Ypsilanti get this work done?

RB: That's an excellent question, and it's not easy. I do find myself saying things to people in positions of power every single day that they don't want to hear, and they don't always react very well to it. It really matters, institution to institution, how you go about it. There are probably a dozen different ways of approaching it. Moving first into a board of directors and acclimating top leadership to these issues is not a bad idea. But, as a young risk manager, you don't always have access to those people. Even I don't have access to those people. Often it takes champions and it takes a lot of champions. You have to have medical people like Skip Campbell who are equally fearless and not defensive. You can chip away at it with the return on investment arguments that are very easy to make. When I said that I started small, that's the first thing that I did. We handled the very first case in a very open way. I took the result of that case, which actually as it turned out the patient decided not only not to bring the claim but asked his lawyer in our presence to stop what he was doing and ask the very doctor we were talking to if he'd take him back as a patient. I told that story in sixty-two speeches that year. I think the stories are important. I think the return on investment analyses are easy to make and important to get out there. I think talking to leadership and making sure that you're not going to get your head handed to you the first time you propose something that sounds crazy is very important, and you've got to have some support. So it's a complex and not always easy thing to do.

RW: You're asking clinicians also to have a new set of skills and probably a new view of their role vis-à-vis patients when there's harm. As you say, part of the pathophysiology of the old system was that something nasty happens and as a doctor I just almost outsource what goes on to somebody else, and now you're asking me to own it, to probably apologize, to sit down with the patient and the family who have been harmed and have difficult conversations to work this thing through. How do you train me to do this so that it doesn't feel like I used to feel, which is that I just sort of want to wash my hands of the whole situation?

RB: I have two responses to that. Let me back up a little bit upstream and say that there's one other thing that I think we need to pay attention to if nationally we're going to move in this direction. I have an advantage that most don't have. I have this luxury to be able to say to a doctor no matter how professionally accountable they need to be, for the outcome that we are confronted with they don't face personal financial ruin. I can't imagine another profession in which the risks are inherent, not completely controllable by the person who might be a defendant in a courtroom, and yet the penalties can seem so draconian. I don't think we're going to fix this until we realize that we need to protect doctors. Hold them accountable but protect them from draconian penalties if we want to protect ultimately our patients and make them safer. That connection is not self-evident to a lot of people, but I think that's absolutely necessary. It's ridiculous to think that a doctor facing potential ruin will come unguarded and talk to the patient about what he or she might have done better and how they might have contributed to the injury. So we have to think about that in those terms.

Secondly, how do you handle this with physicians who may not have been trained to have these difficult conversations? Well, I personally am not an advocate of this notion that you can put somebody through a half a day seminar and then send them out, and in the heat of the moment when it happens to them two or three years later expect that they can handle these things themselves. I think that caregivers are too close, the emotions run too high, and the complex of emotions is too thick. I think they need some help. So even if it's a sole practitioner or someone in a private group just to think about this in advance. Create a relationship with perhaps a lawyer that you trust or somebody else that you trust to be a second set of eyes is absolutely essential. We created a wonderful in-house resource here with risk management that's available 24/7. Every one of our risk managers is a professional trained mediator. We put them through legal mediation training. They're all weathered, highly intelligent, and understand what they're doing. That resource is indispensable to our model. It can be reproduced in a private setting in all sorts of ways. When I was a defense lawyer I would have welcomed a doctor to call me up and say, "Would you be on call if I get into trouble? I just need somebody I trust who understands my ethics and understands what I want to do and can help guide me through this morass."

RW: What does the future hold in this area? Do you see any hope that there will be changes in the overall malpractice system and if so, what would you like to see happen?

RB: In two broad strokes, assuming that we have no changes to our present litigation system what I hope will happen (and I'm seeing this slowly) is that our present way of handling things is driven largely by fear. If we stand for anything, if we can contribute anything to the national dialogue, it should be that one can confront these honestly and with a high degree of accountability and not have the claims sky fall in on them. If we can start to ease the fear a little bit and openly, honestly in these dialogues, then we'll get to the real important point and that is patient safety. Ultimately it's not about claims at all, it's about making people safer. Secondly, in terms of litigation, I am not an advocate at all of the so-called no fault system. Historically tort reforms have meant making it harder to bring claims and making it less lucrative. I think we need to focus on making it less of a game. Right now there's a fundamental flaw in the way we do this. We pick a jury with absolutely no sophistication in these issues, and then we make it a battle of the experts and expect these people we put in the box to know who's telling the truth and who's not. That doesn't make any sense. We need to reinforce the judge's role as a gatekeeper, weed out junk science, make medicine realize that not looking at cases honestly has hurt the whole system, and tighten up expert witness requirements to get rid of the gamesmanship.

RW: Anything else you want to talk about that we haven't covered?

RB: I bristle at the headlines that say apology saves money because ultimately it's not about claims—it's really about patient safety. It's a happy coincidence that apology saves money but it's really about being safer, and that's what I hope to be communicating in this next frontier.

This conversation between two quality of healthcare experts contains sufficient material for several deep discussions, or debates, regarding how to improve the quality of healthcare in America. I consider their conversation to be a very positive contribution toward a safer healthcare system. However, I want to focus on three specific aspects of Mr. Boothman's accomplishment at the University of Michigan Health System over the past decade.

> ***First Point:*** I was overjoyed at Mr. Boothman's reasoning (an experienced trial attorney in medical malpractice matters) in questioning our nation's reliance upon civil litigation as the public's primary system for the review of questionable patient care. Since my first exposure to that system of "Sue or forget it" in the 1970s, I have always felt the same concern. I hope readers will give particular consideration to Mr. Boothman's well-founded disdain for our continuing reliance upon "Sue or forget it" (civil litigation).

Several hundred years ago, it was common practice for doctors to "bleed their patients." Their limited medical understanding in those days left them little choice on how to truly make their patients better. I came to the conclusion many years ago that a similar limited understanding is still in place. The reliance on "Sue or forget it" for the review of questionable patient care has been slowly, and continuously "bleeding" our medical profession of all of the characteristics of a true profession. Until doctors find it within themselves to grow and establish the ability to *fairly judge other doctors* (medical peer review), they will remain a "profession" in name only.

> ***Second Point:*** I thought perhaps that I planted a seed in Dr. Wachter's mind in our brief conversation in 2010 (when I asked him, "How do you get your system of systems errors to every hospital in the nation?"), because late in his conversation with Mr. Boothman, Dr. Wachter asked, "How does the brand-new risk manager at a 150-bed community hospital in Ypsilanti get this work done?"

A better way to ask that question might have been, "How do you get your very positive risk management program to every hospital and surgery center in the State of Michigan?"

Unfortunately, Mr. Boothman could only reply, "That's an excellent question, and it's not easy. I do find myself saying things to people in positions of power every single day that they don't want to hear, and they don't always react very well to it. It really matters, institution to institution, how you go about it."

I believe most of Mr. Boothman's response, as he stated here, is an unintended declaration that there is no organizational structure currently existing in Michigan's state healthcare delivery system, therefore such decisions are left to individual institutions. That doesn't sound very "systematic" to me.

> ***Third Point:*** His comment—"A simple example is a comment that one of our surgeons made to me about two weeks ago. He said to me, 'I was on faculty here six months, at only six months I could give you a short list of people I never wanted to be in an operating room with.' That information is well known. We just need to make greater efforts to tap it and then act on it. Who are those people that everyone knows about who may be unsafe or may be challenged?"

As in most of the literature coming from the quality of healthcare army, an almost complete focus is on systems errors with a correspondingly great absence of consideration for exactly what that surgeon in the quote above was describing to Mr. Boothman (and for what I was forced to act as the second surgeon for in too many cases in Madison, Wisconsin, decades ago). This is my third book on the healthcare delivery system, and I am forced to continue to repeat myself: DOCTORS DON'T KNOW HOW TO JUDGE ONE ANOTHER. They never have, and unfortunately, they have no apparent interest in trying to learn how.

The quality of healthcare army, as demonstrated throughout its literature, appears to have a philosophical aversion to any consideration of individual practitioner patient care negligence. I submit that an estimated 200,000 needless hospital deaths annually cannot be solely due to *systems* errors. Mr. Boothman spoke ever so briefly about "personal accountability or institutional accountability," but, like Dr. Makary in his book *Unaccountable*, neither quality of healthcare expert can describe the source of *authority* that can enable such *accountability* to become meaningful reality.

The previous, positive and informative conversation between two recognized quality of healthcare experts provides a valuable tool for deep consideration regarding several of the many issues weakening the fabric of our healthcare delivery system. Sadly, too few grasp the opportunities this brief article provides. Perhaps as I continue with this exercise in "compare and contrast" such opportunities for deep consideration will become more apparent.

Timeless

Ten years after first seeing, reading, copying, and writing about this next article, I continue to consider it *one of the most important articles in the entire medical literature regarding patient safety*. During my research efforts in 2003 for writing *First, Do No Harm*, I reviewed every issue of the *Journal of American Medical Association (JAMA)* between 1949 and 2003. It continues to amaze me what nuggets one can find in those pages that are ignored and unappreciated.

I included the complete article as it appears in *JAMA* in my first draft of this book, but I was not able to gain permission and that was probably not a good idea to begin with, therefore readers will be limited to my review of that article as written in *Misdiagnosed!*

"Standards for Patient Monitoring During Anesthesia at Harvard Medical School" by John H. Eichhorn, MD; Jeffery B. Cooper, PhD; David J. Cullen, MD; Ward R. Maier, MD; James H. Philip, MD; Robert G. Seeman, MD; JAMA, August 22, 1986.

(*Misdiagnosed! Why Current Healthcare Change is Malpractice* in 2010): Harvard is self-insured and has its own risk management organization.

Even so, Harvard Medical School was not spared as the second wave of the medical malpractice crisis cycled through our nation in the early 1980s. Particularly noteworthy to the Harvard Risk Management Department was the costly impact of the Medical School's Anesthesia Department. That department's leadership was told, "You must do something to greatly improve your present rate of medical liability." To that department's credit, they did do something quick and dramatic. The Harvard Medical School Department of Anesthesia controlled nine separate departments at nine separate hospitals within their system. A committee was formed, and the past patient care incidents were studied to gain an understanding of where the greatest cause(s) of those incidents occurred. Their findings showed that basic patient monitoring practices were thought to be so important in accident prevention that they must become mandatory. The creation of mandatory basic monitoring guidelines in the practice of medicine had never been done before.

The Harvard Medical School Department of Anesthesia devised seven specific, detailed, mandatory standards for minimal patient monitoring during anesthesia at its nine component teaching hospitals. I see those minimal standards like seven lines drawn in the sand that said to every department anesthesiologist, "Doctor, if you cross one of those lines, we cannot help you." By going where no other medical organization had ever gone before, they became professional heretics.

Those seven minimal standards of patient monitoring during anesthesia:

1. Anesthesiologist/nurse anesthetist present in OR
2. Blood pressure and heart rate at five minutes
3. Continuous monitoring (ventilation and circulation)
4. Electrocardiogram
5. Breathing system disconnection monitoring
6. Oxygen analyzer
7. Measure temperature (malignant hyperthermia)

Individually and collectively, none of those minimal standards appear to be asking too much of a dedicated anesthesiologist. Harvard risk management got the quick and dramatic result they were seeking. Within one year, the medical liability rate for that anesthesia department showed a wonderful improvement. But improved quality patient care is not the perspective taken by organized medicine.

Harvard's view of their new, minimum standards: As part of a major patient safety/risk management effort, the Department of Anesthesia of Harvard Medical School, Boston devised specific, detailed, mandatory standards for minimal patient monitoring during anesthesia at its nine component teaching hospitals—*fundamental, minimal standards that would be achievable in the smallest rural community hospital.* Such standards had not previously existed and resistance to the concept was anticipated, but not seen. Physicians have traditionally resisted standards of practice that dictate their day-to-day conduct of medical care.

Organized Medicine's view of those standards: A doctor wrote a fairly lengthy, contrarian response in the same JAMA issue and a small, but insightful excerpt from his review is provided here: "The opportunity for self-determination, for being one's own boss, has been for many of us one of the pluses of being a physician. As such, it is presented not so much t enlighten JAMA readership concerning monitoring as one aspect of anesthesia care, but as an example of a process for extracting a collective minimum standard from individuals long accustomed to defining their own destiny and unaccustomed to others telling them what they should do. The essence of our role as problem-solving givers of care is independent thought and action. Anything that appears to constrain that freedom will be viewed as threatening one's ability to provide care in the way each of us believe to be the best. *We are being provoked to be accountable for both the costs and the benefits of our care.*"

[Too many doctors still think that way and are allowed to conduct their medical practice that way. Where is the medical practice regulatory system?]

My view of those standards: I was taught the first three minimal standards that are noted in the list above in 1963, and the other four minimal standards represent technological advancements. Malignant hyperthermia became a recognized anesthesia hazard in the mid to late 1970s.

Harvard Risk Management view of those standards: No doubt joyful shock at the positive and rapid results of such simple, "mandatory minimums" in patient care and safety.

***Wisconsin State Journal*, December 1986:** A majority of anesthesia deaths are malpractice. As many as 75 percent of the 2,000 or more anesthesia deaths are the result of malpractice. Fourteen percent of 624 cases studied involved failure to maintain the patient's airway open.

Now think about this: In Madison, Wisconsin, in the mid-seventies, a middle-aged wife and mother had a D and C (dilation and curettage procedure) under general anesthesia as the University of Wisconsin hockey team was playing in the NCAA final four on television. *When her anesthesiologist went down the hall to watch the game, her breathing tube disconnected, and she became brain dead.* As Harvard Medical School Department of Anesthesia overview stated, "They are fundamental, minimal standards that would be achievable in the smallest rural community hospital." The above tragedy occurred in the largest hospital in Madison. Now reread organized medicine's response to how those minimal standards were looked at as a threat to the freedom of doing their work as "they thought best." Assume the organization of airline pilots was responding in a like manner to operational restrictions being placed upon their performance. Would such a professional response cause concern from that source?

What if the three Harvard minimal standards of 1986—that I had been taught in 1963—had been minimal standards in every hospital in America during those years? Think of the tragedies that would have been averted by even "three lines in the sand" for all anesthesiologists. That woman in Madison, her family, and her anesthesiologist would not have been forced to face that life-altering event, and that is just one example of what is now euphemistically called *never events.*

Yet after the initial negative response to the original *JAMA* article, and a few additional negative letters to the editor, there was silence from the leaders of organized medicine. There was no bandwagon to jump on. Organized medicine was left with the Harvard Medical School Department of Anesthesia "heretics."

If others view, as I do, the Harvard Anesthesia Department events to be extremely positive steps in patient safety and improved quality of healthcare, then much can be gained from a retrospective study of those events and the responses to them. The initial response from within organized medicine was included in *JAMA.* Far more telling responses can be obtained, if sought.

The Harvard Anesthesia Department event demonstrated rapid and dramatic patient safety improvement by using "a few fundamental, minimal standards that would be achievable in the smallest community hospital." That achievement occurred almost thirty years ago, but there is no evidence it was adopted nationwide. Why not?

Next consider: The Harvard anesthesia example is probably best applied to the other procedure-oriented specialties, but the model is valid for all of American medicine. I define *procedural medicine* to be any type of medical care that pierces the body, i.e., surgery, x-ray therapy, fine-needle biopsies, etc., and in contrast to *diagnostic medicine.*

Harvard School of Public Health has long been a major source of nationally recognized leaders collaborating in the production of volumes of literature related to patient safety and quality healthcare issues. Search the patient safety and quality healthcare literature for any references to the Harvard Anesthesia Department events, but anticipate finding few such references—if any. Positive patient safety efforts ignored should be considered worse than making no efforts whatsoever to improve patient safety.

Quality of healthcare offerings provide models for improving patient safety using guidelines and standards formulated by experts far removed from the site of questionable patient care and utilizing "systems cures" based within "non-punitive environments." Apparently when individual doctors harm patients, those issues are abandoned to that Faustian bargain that left both doctors and the public with the adversarial system that Mr. Boothman referred to, and that I call "Sue or forget it."

A system of hospital medical staff peer review presented later in this book is based upon doctors fairly judging other doctors rapidly and at the site of the questionable patient care. Harvard Anesthesia Department long ago proved the dramatic value of such a patient safety reform while using only a very few minimum standards.

Patient safety activists should ask themselves, "Which method of improved patient safety best offers the quality healthcare changes I am seeking at the hospital medical staff nearest me?"

Perhaps even more distressing should be the scarcity of positive patient safety events to be found in the medical literature. The Harvard Medical School Department of Anesthesia minimum standards with their rapid and greatly beneficial result should have been a beacon of light in the quest for greater patient safety. Try to find those who have even heard about it enough to retain its value.

All healthcare is local, and the Harvard Anesthesia Department *proved* that the regulation of medical practice applied at the local level could provide the most rapid and effective results. Compare the Harvard results to the current healthcare cottage industry results of sanctimonious, nonspecific guidelines for greater patient safety that in ten years have yielded no evidence of benefit to society at the hospital medical staff level of the hospital nearest you.

Authority, responsibility, and most important of all, accountability, must function within every hospital medical staff in the nation, but those critical elements must have a clearly defined organizational structure before they can function properly. Far too many people continue to die needlessly in our hospitals in spite of monumental efforts by so many, while everyone continues to look for solutions that are meant to "trickle down from on high."

What did the Harvard Anesthesia Minimum Standard Really Demonstrate? Organized Structure, Authority, and Delegated Authority

I wrote most of the above assessment of the Harvard Medical School Department of Anesthesia minimum standards in 2009, before my offer to Governor Haley, Dr. Makary's book *Unaccountable* and my belated recognition of the accountability equation. I speak of those elements in my assessment, but I was never able to fully appreciate their combined impact until I related Dr. Makary's strong emphasis on accountability and my Air Force delegated authority over fifty years ago.

July 1, 1963, I began my three-year oral and maxillofacial surgery residency in Milwaukee, Wisconsin, in a VA/Marquette University, Medical College of Wisconsin joint program. I began my residency with a six-month rotation on anesthesia at Milwaukee County Hospital and in a program chaired by Dr. Jay Jacoby. Under his training I was able to do several spinals and a few subdural (saddle blocks), plus great training in blind intubations.

Dr. Jacoby learned anesthesia in an on-the-job training program in mash units during WWII in Europe. He said, when combat circumstances demanded, he got to where he stood like a center pole and provided ether anesthesia for up to four surgical cases at a time. There's good, and then there is really GOOD.

Dr. Jacoby returned and created the first Department of Anesthesia at Ohio State University in 1947. He is credited with instituting the use of recovery rooms, ICUs, "Code Blue," and many other cutting-edge anesthesia advancements. When I began to write *First, Do No Harm* in 2003, I made a point of tracking him down. He had recently retired to South Florida after fifty-eight years of teaching anesthesia to doctors, oral surgeons, and nurses at three separate institutions. I told him I was beginning to write a book on medical malpractice. He said he had been thinking about doing the same. I said we need to get together, and I thought about making a trip South. Several weeks later a son-in-law called to inform me that Dr. Jacoby had died suddenly.

There can never be too many Jay Jacobys.

Back to this chapter's beginning . . . .

Just using the two articles featured in this chapter, I could spend several days teaching a class of young people who think they want to spend their life becoming quality of healthcare experts. So many of the elements of quality of patient care issues are touched on and passively left for another day or for someone else to address.

That surgeon told Mr. Boothman that in only six months he was able to identify several "problematic surgeons" on that medical center's surgical staff, but he would not provide names. I learned the hard way that you don't break the code of silence. Yet no one within the quality of healthcare army can tell how to identify problematic practitioners in a fair manner. I can provide a system of medical peer review that could fairly judge the questionable care of another practitioner, but the quality of healthcare army is apparently too focused on systems errors.

Peter Pronovost, MD, PhD [permission granted]

Dr. Pronovost is a practicing anesthesiologist and critical care physician, teacher, researcher, and international patient safety leader. He is a professor in the Johns Hopkins University School of Medicine (departments of Anesthesiology and Critical Care Medicine, and Surgery) in the Bloomberg School of Public Health (Department of Health Policy and Management) and in the School of Nursing. He is also medical director for the Center for Innovation and Quality Patient Care, which supports quality and safety efforts at the Johns Hopkins hospitals. In 2003 Dr. Pronovost established the Quality and Safety Research Group to advance the science of safety. Dr. Pronovost and his research team are dedicated to improving healthcare through methods that are scientifically rigorous, but feasible at the bedside. Dr. Pronovost holds a doctorate in clinical investigation from the Johns Hopkins Bloomberg School of Public Health.

Dr. Pronovost chairs the JCAHO ICU Advisory Panel for Quality Measures, the ICU Physician Staffing Committee for the Leapfrog Group, and serves on the Quality Measures Work Group of the National Quality Forum. He also serves in an advisory capacity to the World Health Organizations World Alliance for Patient Safety, and is leading WHO efforts to improve patient safety measurement, evaluation, and leadership capacity globally.

Time magazine, in 2008, named Dr. Pronovost one of the world's most influential people for his work in patient safety. The magazine's annual list recognizes people "whose power, talent or moral example is transforming our world." Dr. Pronovost also received the MacArthur Foundation Fellowship, commonly known as a "genius grant" in 2008.

The Pronovost Checklist

Central venous catheters, or lines, are used for medications, blood, fluids or nutrition and can stay in for days or weeks. But bacteria can grow in the line and spread a type of infection to the bloodstream, which causes death in one out of five patients who contract it. This five-step checklist for doctors and nurses to use before inserting a line can prevent infections and death.

1. Wash hands with soap and water or an alcohol cleanser.
2. Wear sterile clothing—a mask, gloves, and hair covering—and cover patient with a sterile drape, except for a very small hole where the line goes in.
3. Clean patient's skin with chlorhexidine (a type of soap) when the line is put in.
4. Avoid veins in arm and leg, which are more likely to get infected than veins in chest.
5. Check the line for infection each day, and remove when no longer needed.

In "The Secret to Fighting Infections" Dr. Pronovost says it isn't that hard, If only hospitals would do it. Laura Landro, in a WSJ interview asked Dr. Pronovost, "In your book you describe how hard it is to bring innovation and change to hospitals. What are the barriers to innovation?"

Excerpts from Dr. Pronovost's Responses

"The main barriers are the lack of collaboration and a culture that is resistant to change. There is also a lack of systems integration."

"In healthcare we need leadership to create a partnership between academic medicine and industry to pilot-test a new model."

"The pilot who neglects a checklist before takeoff would not be allowed to fly, and most safe industries have transgressions that are firing offenses. But there hasn't been that kind of accountability in healthcare."

"But physicians are often self-employed, have little training in teamwork and perhaps like all of us, are often overconfident about the quality of care they provide, believing things will go right rather than wrong."

"Medicare provides a lot of money for training programs, and the federal government could require that we produce doctors in this country who are better trained in teamwork."

"The Department of Health and Human Services has called for a 50 percent reduction in central line blood stream infections over three years, but in some states only 20 percent of hospitals have signed up."

"What is perhaps most concerning is when I asked nurses, 'If you saw a senior physician not comply with the checklist, would you speak up and would the physician comply?' Uniformly, the answer is no."

"We have the knowledge about how to prevent infections, but it is just not being used or getting the attention it deserves, and that is just astounding."

Read again Dr. Pronovost's "main barriers impeding positive change":

- A culture that is resistant
- A lack of leadership to create partnerships
- A lack of accountability
- A lack of teamwork training

Now I ask, "What seems to be missing in his list of barriers to innovation?"

Dr. Atul Gawande [Dr. Gawande's speakers bureau profile] [permission granted]

This professor at Harvard Medical School, and best-selling author of The Checklist Manifesto is the physician's physician – the definitive voice on improving healthcare.

> "Dr. Gawande's bold visions for improving performance and safety in healthcare have made him one of the most sought-after speakers in medicine. *TIME* placed him among the world's 100 most influential thinkers. He is a MacArthur "Genius" Fellowship winner in 2006, a *New Yorker* columnist, and author—but, most of all, a physician, with a practitioners grasp of the everyday challenges of healthcare delivery.
>
> "Dr. Gawande explains that medical practice and philosophy has not kept pace with the changes in healthcare over the last hundred years. We need reform—and Dr. Gawande is on a lifelong search to discover what shape that reform should take. What does an effective healthcare system look like in the twenty-first century? How can we improve quality, manage risk, and measure performance more effectively? Dr. Gawande brings an eloquence and an intellect to these questions that allow him to offer deeply considered and beautifully express solutions with implications for healthcare and beyond.
>
> "He is broadly known for his influential articles, two of which won him the National Magazine Award. He has written about the shift from lone-ranger physicians to teams of cooperating specialists, and the new values this shift requires. He popularized the checklist as a means of coordinating complex work in hospitals. His ideas about how to rein in healthcare cost while increasing efficiency and quality have transformed the national discussion of these issues. His writing sets itself apart by its depth of thought and research, but also by its willingness to look outside of healthcare and see how other fields have delivered high quality service in complex industries.
>
> "Dr. Gawande practices general and endocrine surgery at Brigham and Women's Hospital in Boston. He is also a professor of Surgery at Harvard Medical School and professor at the Harvard School of Public Health. He is the head of Ariadne Labs, a joint center for health systems innovation created with Brigham and Women's Hospital and the Harvard School of Public Health. Dr. Gawande serves as lead advisor for the World Health Organization's Safe Surgery

Saves Lives program, and is the founding chairman of Lifebox, an international not-for- profit implementing systems and technologies to reduce surgical deaths globally. He is one of *Foreign Policy*'s top 100 influential Thinkers, and the winner of AcademyHealth's Impact Award for highest research impact on healthcare."

Keywords for Dr. Gawande as a speaker include: burning issues, checklist, columnists, ethics and values, healthcare reform, MacArthur Fellowship, medical ethics, patient care, patient safety, risk, science, and storytelling.

South Carolina Hospital Association News announced September 17, 2010 "South Carolina Chosen as Pilot for National Effort to Improve Surgical Safety: Efforts expected to reduce patient deaths by hundreds each year."

The South Carolina Hospital Association is embarking on a new patient safety program that can potentially save hundreds of patient lives each year and reduce the number of major surgical complications up to 30 percent. South Carolina is partnering with renowned surgeon and author, Dr. Gawande, in introducing a Surgical Safety Checklist in every operating room in the state.

Dr. Gawande currently serves as the lead of the World Health Organization's Safe Surgery Saves Lives initiative where they created a three-part surgical checklist that was demonstrated to reduce surgery related complications by more than one-third. Most recently, Dr. Gawande documented his experience creating and testing the WHO Surgical Safety Checklist in his *New York Times* bestseller, *The Checklist Manifesto*.

"We selected South Carolina to be the first state to partner with us to help improve surgical safety around the entire country," said Dr. Gawande. "South Carolina has a tremendous history of successfully introducing other quality initiatives such as improving the care of heart attack patients and reducing infection. South Carolina hospitals have already demonstrated their commitment to improving surgical safety by initially testing the World Health Organization's Surgical Safety Checklist in more than 80 percent of the state's hospitals, many of which have since adopted the checklist as a routine component of surgical care. We would like to collaborate with South Carolina hospitals in developing a model to improve surgical safety at a state level that other US states can follow." South Carolina was recently ranked by the federal government as one of five states making the most improvements in the quality and safety of healthcare. "We want to be the safest state and have the highest quality of care. That's our vision," said Dr. Rick Foster, SCHA senior vice president for quality and patient safety. "These numbers are an indication of our success. And working with Dr. Gawande is a tremendous opportunity to lead the nation in improving surgical safety." In January 2009 the results of an international multi-center pilot study measuring the impact of the World Health Organization's Surgical Safety Checklist were published in the *New England Journal of Medicine.* This study demonstrated that by using a simple nineteen-item checklist the rate of major complications following surgery fell from 11 percent in the baseline to 7 percent after an introduction of the checklist. Inpatient deaths following major operations fell by more than 40 percent (from 1.5 percent to 0.8 percent). The nineteen actions listed on the checklist include making sure antibiotics were given within the past sixty minutes, marking the surgical site, setting aside blood, verifying the patient's identity, and having all members of the surgical team introduce themselves. While these may sound like common sense, one or more can be overlooked and often are, judging from the number of surgical complications and deaths each year.

With more than 700,000 surgeries performed annually in South Carolina the introduction and proper use of a surgical checklist could greatly impact the number of complications that surgical patients may suffer from and prevent hundreds of patients from dying each year.

Yet, only 20 percent of American hospitals are following the checklist, and Dr. Gawande is determined to change that, starting with South Carolina. The goal of the partnership with South Carolina is to introduce a checklist in every hospital and have it used for every surgical patient. Using the best practices identified in the lessons learned in South Carolina, he plans ultimately to take the surgical safety program to other states.

"We are thrilled that South Carolina has been selected as the lead state because of our commitment to quality and patient safety and the success we've experience," said SCHA President and CEO Thornton Kirby. "Using the best practices identified and the lessons learned in South Carolina, Dr. Gawande plans ultimately to take the surgical safety program to other states."

Dr. Gawande's interview with the *Greenville News* provided these additional comments:
"Surgical complications injure and kill thousands of people in the Palmetto State every year but many could be saved if hospitals used a simple safety checklist."

"The average hospital has a serious surgical complication rate of 3 percent said Dr. Gawande."

"I do about 300 operations a year and that means I have about ten patients I seriously harm," he said. "And at least half the time the harm was avoidable."

Checklists Save Lives

I learned the value of a checklist long before Doctors Gawande and Pronovost were born, and I support the positive value of checklists in our healthcare delivery system (every hospital and surgery center). But I feel I must critique some of the shortcomings that are clearly evident to me in their efforts to improve the quality and safety of healthcare and how limited those efforts will continue to be within our current, unorganized, and dysfunctional healthcare delivery system.

First, more about the military aviation checklist, and how many unknown number of times they probably saved my life.

I began using checklists in combat military aircraft in South Korea in 1954. 17th Bomb Wing had three squadrons that flew WWII twin-engine medium bombers that had two configurations. Most planes had a glass nose and a crew of four: pilot in the left seat, flight engineer in the right seat, a tail gunner, and me forward in the glass nose as the navigator-bombardier with the Norden bombsight. The hard-nose configuration required a three-man crew, pilot, gunner, and me in the right seat as the navigator-flight engineer. That hard nose contained one 37 mm cannon and three 50 caliber machine guns. My job on strafing training missions was to pat the pilot's right shoulder as he approached the altitude to begin his pullout, and to beat him on his shoulder if and when he began to go beyond that level. Pilots have been known to become so fixated that they flew into the ground, or the Sea of Japan south of Korea in our case.

Every flight required step-by-step use of the checklist from the moment we entered the plane until the engine shut down, and this familiarity with the importance of checklist would lead me into creating my offer of an Individual Responsibility Peer Review system checklist that goes far beyond those checklists offered by Doctors Gawande and Pronovost. More on that later.

After our Bomb Wing transferred from K-9 Pusan Korea due east, across the Sea of Japan to Miho AFB on the North shore of the main Japanese Island, and due north of Hiroshima, our training missions became longer. On hard-nose training flights, we were occasionally forced to land for refueling at Fukuoka AFB, located south of Miho and about equidistant between Hiroshima and Nagasaki. As navigator-engineer, I stood on top of the wings and refueled both tanks for our return flight home. Therefore, when I trained and later used my private pilot's license, while training to become a board-certified oral surgeon, and while stilling flying with the Wisconsin Air National Guard, the use of checklist was well ingrained into my psyche.

Checklist Critique

Dr. Gawande received his MacArthur "genius award" in 2006, and Dr. Pronovost received that same award in 2008 (some feel those award recognitions should have been in reverse order, but both are well deserved). As both safety experts will admit, their greatest problem is getting those safety improvements to become uniformly used throughout every hospital (and hopefully every surgery center) in the nation.

Why? Both doctors have given multiple, vague reasons, i.e., "lack of collaboration and a culture that is 'resistant' to change," or "there hasn't been that kind of 'accountability' in healthcare," etc.

I believe there are, and have always been, those three key words missing in our nation's healthcare delivery system. What would a healthcare system look like, and how would it function IF it had an organizational structure, with clearly defined points of *authority,* and *delegated authority* sufficiently able to create meaningful *accountability*? Different!

Doctors Gawande and Pronovost cannot provide detailed information on how well their very positive and very beneficial safety efforts have become as consistently routine as the use of checklists in Air Force aircraft, because the military has what our nation's healthcare delivery system does not have, and has always needed.

Case in point: SCHA News Release September 17, 2010

"South Carolina hospitals have already demonstrated their commitment to improving surgical safety by initially testing the World Health Organization's Surgical Safety Checklist *in more than 80 percent of the state's hospitals, many of which have since adopted the checklist as a routine component of surgical care*" (emphasis added).

South Carolina Hospital Association has been "testing the Surgical Safety Checklist in *less than 100 percent of the state's hospitals,* because SCHA is an *association*, therefore they *have no authority over their members* and *not all South Carolina hospitals are members of SCHA*. One of the major points that would have been provided by Phase 1 of my offer to Governor Haley and the SC Legislative members I met with is the facts about what SCHA, and every other component of that state's healthcare delivery system can and cannot do, in spite of everything they have long been saying about what they have been doing, and while so many people are continuing to die needlessly in this, and every other state's hospitals.

Another case in point: NO member of the army of quality of healthcare experts has AUTHORITY that can be directly utilized in any hospital or surgery center in America. The best Doctors Gawande and Pronovost and the countless others like them can do is to ask the doctors of America, "PLEASE!"

The ability to practice medicine is a privilege provided by a state license. Doctors have always treated that privilege as though it was their birthright, and states have permitted them to do so.

HOSPITAL (AND SURGERY CENTERS) CONTINUE TO BE THE ONLY PLACES IN AMERICA WHERE ACCIDENTAL DEATH RECEIVES NO IMMEDIATE REVIEW BY A STATE SOURCE OF AUTHORITY.

Additional thoughts regarding Drs. Gawande, Pronovost and Wachter

On September 17, 2010, a South Carolina Hospital Association press release regarding their collaboration with Dr. Gawande and his checklist method for patient safety appeared.

On September 30, 2010, Dr. Wachter's presentation and our brief conversation occurred, and later our exchange of emails where he thought my book, *Misdiagnosed*, about which he said it "made some important points and I agree that peer review is a critical, and mostly neglected component of patient safety."

That South Carolina Hospital Association press release and my email exchange with Dr. Wachter led me to contact Dr. Gawande, also by email, where I suggested we exchange signed copies of our books.

I received the following message though his assistant: "Thank you for offering to send Dr. Gawande a book. He wishes he could send you a signed copy, but we have been out of books since January! He asked me to let you know that he'll file your email for future visits to South Carolina. He hopes someday he'll be able to meet with you."

I sent Dr. Gawande a signed copy of *Misdiagnosed* with the following letter enclosed:

Dr. Gawande,

With the utmost courtesy and respect, I feel the efforts of the last twenty years to greatly improve the quality of healthcare in general and medical care specifically have been misdirected. Furthermore, I believe there is an abundance of proof evident, but largely ignored, to support that premise.

Even more remarkable is the reluctance of those seeking to improve the healthcare system to participate, or even allow, an open discussion on why the tragic rate of needless hospital deaths continues to increase in spite of all of the efforts of an army of healthcare experts' endeavors to reverse that trend.

I was delighted to see the South Carolina Hospital Association announcement that you had selected South Carolina as the pilot for a national effort to improve surgical safety. Hopefully this will provide an opportunity to compare our use of the checklist for providing greater patient safety.

I have over 2,700 hours as an Air Force navigator- bombardier; I am a licensed pilot (single-engine) and have flown a glider from takeoff to landing. In 1970, I, acting alone, organized the first surgical mini-residency for the surgical correction of jaw deformities in Madison, Wisconsin. The second such surgical mini-residency was held at Dallas Parkland Hospital and the third at their sister program in Fort Worth.

As I told Dr. Robert Wachter during his recent visit to Greenville, I feel I am fully qualified to participate in helping to make our healthcare system far better and am as passionate about wishing to contribute is any other person. I do hope the Big Tent for Better Patient Care you are helping to erect in South Carolina will permit me to enter and contribute.

Sincerell.y,
Dr. Ira Williams

Both Dr. Gawande and Dr. Wachter were back in South Carolina at the invitation of the South Carolina Hospital Association early in 2011, but I am yet to hear from either patient safety expert.

Dr. Gawande's interview with the *Greenville News* led to this interesting comment: "I do about 300 operations a year, and that means I have about ten patients I seriously harm," he said. "And at least half the time, the harm was avoidable."

Brigham and Women's Hospital in Boston must have a fantastic risk management system that must rival the one Mr. Boothman has established at the University of Michigan Medical Center. With numerous operating rooms going seven days a week and hundreds of surgeons, if one of the best surgeons in the country has such a consistent patient safety record, the risk management people must really be busy. Twenty-five injured patients due to avoidable harm in five years by the same surgeon should rapidly increase that surgeon's awareness for increased patient safety improvement. Would his airline have continued to allow Sully to keep flying passengers across the country if he had been averaging five hard landings that caused airplane damage each year? Those who desperately want to include more airline safety measures into the practice of medicine clearly have their work cut out for them.

But there is more:

Balancing "No Blame" with Accountability in Patient Safety, Robert M. Wachter, MD, and Peter J. Pronovost, MD., PhD. NEJM, October 1, 2009.

["Stop the blame game – most medical errors are systems errors" has long been the mantra of the quality of healthcare army of experts, even though most second surgeons are ask to repair other doctor's errors (I speak from experience). In this article two of the most nationally recognized patient safety experts attempt to walk a very fine line between two realities, "no blame" falls far short of its target and there is little, if any real progress being made in making patient care truly safer, in spite of all of the effort by that enormous army of quality of healthcare experts.]

It takes the authors four and a half pages of text and 33 references in their attempt to find an equitable balance when discussing "no blame" versus accountability. They recognize that regulators out-side the medical profession may equate the "no blame" approach as an example of guild behavior (which it is). Their conclusion, if one can call it that, is that there does come a time when their profession *must deem certain behaviors as unacceptable*, with clear consequences in order to illustrate their true professionalism.

The entire article takes literary license to an extreme and creates far more questions that are passively ignored than clear answers being provided. But what is the specific patient safety issue that can cause two patient safety experts to openly question "no blame"?

Hand Hygiene

The above article offers Table 1: Prerequisites for Making the Choice to Punish Providers for Not Adhering to a Patient-Safety Practice, Using the Example of hand hygiene.

Mr. Boothman was told by a surgeon that he was only on that medical staff six months and had identified several surgeons of highly questionable surgical expertise. I predict that

Mr. Boothman still cannot identify who those surgeons are to this day. People wonder why the needless hospital death rate is higher and going in the wrong direction. Now, reread their article while knowing that *hand hygiene* is the focal point of the need to better balance practitioner accountability with patient-safety practices.

Hand hygiene is important and can save lives, just as Doctors Gawande and Pronovost checklists can save lives. But in *First, Do No Harm* (2004) and in its very positive *New England Journal of Medicine* review I said I could provide a system of medical peer review, much more fair to both doctor and patient, based on a checklist and the individual doctor's patient care track record, and not just one isolated incident. I am still waiting on Drs. Gawande and Wachter to get back to me.

One last bone to pick with Drs. Gawande and Wachter

Both Dr. Gawande and Dr. Wachter really got under my skin when, on separate occasions, they chose to denigrate the integrity of arguably the greatest pilot in the history of the Air Force, Chuck Yeager.

Dr. Gawande, in *The Checklist Manifesto* had this to say: "Tom Wolfe's *The Right Stuff* tells the story of our first astronauts and charts the demise of the maverick, Chuck Yeager test pilot culture of the 1950s. It was a culture defined by how unbelievably dangerous the job was. Test pilots strapped themselves into machines of barely controlled power and complexity, and a quarter of them were killed on the job. The pilots had to have focus, daring, wits, and an ability to improvise – the right stuff. But as knowledge of how to control the risk of flying accumulated – as checklists and flight simulators became more prevalent and sophisticated – the danger diminished, values of safety and conscientiousness prevailed, and the rock star status of the test pilot was gone.

Dr. Wachter, in his September 2010 presentation at Greenville Memorial Hospital, closed his remarks by making a far more disparaging characterization of Chuck Yeager, himself, and I immediately took vocal, but muted exception to his slander of a person, still living, who deserves better, from everyone.

Some people's mavericks are other people's heroes. I happened to have had an opportunity to play a very minor part in that early era of pushing that envelope in the sky, and I loved it. My South Korea-Japan unit island- hopped our WWII planes back across the Pacific in early 1955 to our new base, Eglin #9, Hulbert AFB, Florida. That summer we transitioned into jet engine medium bombers and I found myself flying at 50,000 ft., where the blue turns black, on the edge of space. During my first flight at that level, my pilot and I were able to circle the stalk of a Texas thunderstorm while looking up to its anvil-shaped top, probably at 80,000–85,000 feet. They called that pushing the envelope, and for a twenty-two-year-old it was as close to heaven as I had been thus far. On one clear winter night flight at that level out of Blytheville AFB I could turn my head from right to left and identify the lights of St. Louis, Kansas City, Topeka, Wichita, Tulsa, and the glow of Oklahoma City. As we turned to return home, Milwaukee and Chicago appeared to be connected by a row of streetlights. Little did I know then that I would spend three years of my life in Milwaukee beginning seven years later, in 1963.

So let me describe a few "mavericks" in healthcare.

Dr. Wachter momentarily shocked me when he began his presentation here in Greenville, South Carolina, by mentioning, very briefly, Dr. Semmelweis, who first pioneered the need for doctors to wash both their hands and instruments. My shock was due to the fact that the medical profession cannot be proud of the full story of Semmelweis even today.

But I believe the Semmelweis story is important.

Dr. Ignaz Semmelweis (maverick) 1818–1865

Semmelweis was a Hungarian physician who was employed as an assistant to the professor of the maternity clinic at the Vienna General Hospital in Austria in 1847. During that year he noticed that a close friend of his had cut his finger while he was doing an autopsy, and that friend soon died of symptoms like that of puerperal fever.

That event caused Semmelweis to connect two disparate epidemiological facts: the death rate at his hospital of women who gave birth was 13 percent, and at a nearby hospital run by midwives their death rate was 2 percent. He also had observed that medical students were going from the anatomical dissection room to the delivery room without changing their outer garments or washing their hands.

These observations led Semmelweis to become a medical maverick. He began a study that first merely caused doctors to wash their hands in a chlorine solution when they left the anatomical dissection room. The mortality rate from puerperal fever rapidly dropped to 2 percent. However instead of reporting his success at a meeting, Semmelweis said nothing. Finally a friend published two papers on the method, but by that time Semmelweis had started washing medical instruments as well as their hands.

The hospital director felt his leadership had been criticized by Semmelweis's studies, and he was furious. He blocked Semmelweis's promotion and the situation continued to deteriorate. Viennese doctors turned on their Hungarian maverick. The medical leaders in Vienna said that IF they were to accept his findings and his methods, they would be forced to admit that they, and their now recognized outdated patient care methods were, and long had been, the cause of their much higher death rate. That they would never do, in spite of his overwhelming evidence in greater patient safety.

Facing rejection by his medical colleagues in Vienna, he returned to Budapest; and there he brought his methods to a far more primitive hospital. Those methods allowed him to cut the death rate by puerperal fever to less than 1 percent. He continued to expand his studies into the need for greater hygiene by physicians until finally, in 1861, he wrote a book on his methods. However the medical community in Budapest was no more receptive then his colleagues in Vienna had been. His book and his methods were given poor reviews, and his response unfortunately grew from anger into rage and frustration.

In 1865 he suffered a mental breakdown and friends committed him to a mental institution. There, he ended his brief forty-seven-year life by cutting his finger and within days he died of the very infection that had killed his friend previously and from what he'd saved thousands of mothers.

Joseph Lister (1827–1912)

The "Father of Antiseptic Surgery" gained the attention Semmelweis earned and deserved, but Lister always acknowledged that he had stood on the shoulders of a Hungarian doctor who had been vilified by the leadership of the profession he had so loved and sought to serve.

The full details of Semmelweis, his contributions, and his complete rejection by his profession's leadership is not a story one can expect to hear at a medical presentation.

Sir John Dr. Charnley (another maverick) (1911–1982)

Dr. Charnley was the father of the total hip procedure. He became a fellow of the Royal College of Surgeons in England in 1936. In May 1940 he volunteered for army service, entering the Royal Army Medical Corps as a lieutenant, then he was promoted to major. His postings included Northern Ireland, the Middle East, and the evacuation of Dunkirk.

In 1958 Dr. Charnley decided to put his efforts into the development of hip replacement research and surgery. For the next several years he suffered trial and tribulations when developing his hip replacement, but he never gave up. Finally in November 1962 the Charnley hip replacement became practical reality and has become the gold standard for this form of treatment.

Dr. Charley's total hip replacement procedure was probably the first modern surgical procedure to not only treat a patient's major problem but to also improve the quality of life following that procedure. Thus the total hip replacement procedure that is so common today has recently celebrated its fiftieth anniversary. Dr. Charnley also developed the concept of laminar airflow to eradicate a systemic infection problem in his hospital.

Side note: In the mid-1970s, thanks to the effort of a mutual friend, I had an opportunity to enjoy Sunday dinner at the English estate of a former commodore of the London Yacht Club. While admiring a picture of his yacht that he and his family used for routine sailing in the Mediterranean and elsewhere, I happened to ask him, "Were you at Dunkirk?" He simply replied, "Yes."

Am I a maverick?

In the mid-1960s the surgical correction of jaw deformities began to open like time-lapsed photos of a flower opening. During my three-year surgical residency that ended in 1966, I had not had an opportunity to be trained in those types of procedures. An editorial in the

Journal of Oral Surgery in the fall of 1969 spoke of the need for surgical mini-residencies; and upon reading that I said, "That's exactly what I need."

But I knew that my best opportunity for such a mini-residency experience would only come about if I organized such an event myself. I also realized that to do that, I would have to:

1. Find a dual-degree surgeon who would be willing to conduct such an event.
2. Find sufficient patients who would need such certain surgical correction.
3. Find a sufficient number of practicing oral surgeons who would be willing to attend such an event and help cover the cost.

One afternoon I went to the State Board of Medical Examiners and provided them with information regarding an MD/DDS chairman of Oral Surgery at the University of Texas/Houston. I was informed that it would be no problem for them to grant that person or someone with similar credentials a temporary Wisconsin medical license in order to conduct such a mini-residency event.

That same afternoon, I met with the administrator of the smallest of the three private hospitals and asked him if such an event would be feasible at their facility. He assured me that they would gladly give me complete support for such an event, including operating room scheduling and lecture room accommodations.

In early 1970 I took and successfully passed the certification process to become a diplomat of the American Board of Oral and Maxillofacial Surgery. Shortly after that, I was able to visit Houston and layout my plan for the late Dr. Edward Hinds. His response was that he was very willing to participate in such an event, but assumed it would take a year or more to bring everything together. I told Dr. Hinds that my target date was for June of that year, but we would both see how things progressed.

In June 1970 the first mini-residency for the surgical correction of jaw deformities took place in Madison, Wisconsin. Oral surgeons from five states attended that week-long mini-residency where eight patients were operated on during the first four days in the mornings, and we then met with Dr. Hinds in the afternoons. Friday of that week was used for follow-up of all the proceeding surgeries and a final dinner.

The second mini-residency for the surgical correction of jaw deformities took place at Parkland Hospital Dallas, Texas, a couple of years later, followed by a similar mini-residency at their sister oral surgery program in Fort Worth. Those two hospitals continued a series of mini-residencies for several years, and several other oral surgery teaching programs held similar events.

Semmelweis's story is not, unfortunately, a rare occurrence throughout the history of medicine. Such rejection of offerings that go counter to the current norms within that profession decorate the history of learned men seeking to improve their healing methods.

Doctors Gawande and Wachter both accepted copies of my book, *Misdiagnosed*, and I presume Dr. Gawande read it, as Dr. Wachter said he did. But their reading my book happened after Dr. Wachter told me that "their attempts to get their patient care improvements to every hospital in America was a 'problem,'" and I said I can solve that problem, and he said *nothing*. Now those two nationally recognized quality of healthcare experts have been joined by another, equally recognized, and deservedly so, person seeking to make healthcare in America far better.

Sully and a New Federal Bureaucracy

Sully Sullenberger has joined forces with three other notables in their own right seeking a major new federal bureaucracy to join in the effort to make healthcare safer. That combination of national hero and laudable cause should make their call for action immune from challenge. But challenge them I do, confident that the Sully the nation now knows will be willing to honor one of the closing remarks in their thoughtful paper: "It is time for civil debate, real solutions, and authentic governing."

I say, let the debate begin. Just tell me where and when. I only ask for equal time and equal courtesy.

As will be described in some detail in the next chapter there have been efforts to create a bureaucratic process to confront patient care problems during the past several decades, and those efforts have all met with failure. What is not discussed in the depth it should be are the multiple reasons why those efforts inevitably will lead to failure. People continue to try to make the quality of healthcare better from the top down, but their efforts are denied the necessary mechanism to make those efforts become reality where the rubber meets the road in healthcare, at the doctor/patient interface, and in every hospital and surgery center in the nation.

But first let's take a bit-by-bit look at the proposal offered by Sully and his equally qualified cohorts as it appeared in the *Journal of Patient Safety* in March 2012.

"An NTSB for healthcare – Learning from Innovation: Debate and Innovate or Capitulate" was written by Charles R. Denham, MD, Chesley B. Sullenberger, III, MS, Dennis W. Quaid, and John J. Nance, JD.

Dr. Charles Denham is the chairman Texas Medical Institute of Technology and editor of the *Journal of Patient Safety,* and much, much, more. Sully Sullenberger should need no further introduction, I assume. Actor Dennis Quaid likewise should need no further introduction. John Nance is a former military and commercial pilot, author, and also much more.

All four men have been jet pilots, two both in the military and airlines. The three non-physicians have been drawn to the problems within our healthcare system by real, and in the case of Dennis Quaid, all-too-real healthcare events in their lives. Their ardor for their cause cannot be questioned. But I will first offer a brief description of the federal agency they feel offers a perfect model for what is needed in healthcare. Regretfully, none of these thumbnail descriptions do those individuals the justice they each deserve, but the hope is that this brief review will spur some, perhaps many, to take a long, hard look at their "proposed" new federal bureaucracy.

National Transportation Safety Board (NTSB)

NTSB investigations cover four separate areas: Aviation, Highway, Marine, and Railroad, Pipeline, and Hazardous Materials.

- The Board investigates about 2,000 aviation accidents and incidents a year, and about 500 accidents in the other modes of transportation—rail, highway, marine, and pipeline.
- The Safety Board has no regulatory or enforcement powers.
- To ensure that Safety Board investigations focus only on improving transportation safety, the Board's analysis of factual information and its determination of probable cause cannot be entered as evidence in a court of law.
- Safety recommendations are the most important part of the Safety Board's mandate.

A review of the Denham, Sully, Quaid, Nance proposal hopefully will be more revealing with the above sketch of the current NTSB.

Now back to An NTSB for Healthcare: [Note: The article contains nine pages of text and two and a half pages with 85 references. I have requested copyright permission to use about two-dozen brief excerpts, with my responses, from Dr. Denham, Editor-in-Chief of the Journal of Patient Safety, but my permission request has received no response. Strange behavior from those seeking "civil debate", thus the need to paraphrase.]

The four aviators indicate in the introduction that this will be the first of a two-part paper recognizing the need for and the benefits of a healthcare clone of the National Transportation Safety Board (NTSB) and their quest to seek a debate for such. Also reference to the planned scope of their promised Part II article was included.

My response: The need for such a debate is long overdue.

The authors collectively offer assurance that their knowledge and understanding of aviation and the benefits of the NTSB can rapidly translate into saving lives and money throughout our nation's healthcare system.

My response: Meaningful change based upon theoretical promises all too often fail to fulfill those promises, thus the great need for the open debate they claim to desire.

The authors recognize the extreme magnitude of needless hospital deaths, and refer to the World Health Organization (WHO) biased and negative evaluation of our current healthcare system, and how even those states that seem to focus on patient safety continue to fall far short.

My response: That first sentence is an indictment of the past twenty years of quality of healthcare army's unproductive efforts. I reject the World Health Organization's specious ranking of our healthcare system as being 37th in the world. WHO downgrades our healthcare system simply because we do not have their desired system of a governmentally controlled system. The last portion of that statement describes a major part of the premise of this book.

The authors emphasis the similarities between the delivery of healthcare and passengers to their destinations both depend upon reliable human performance, but only if basic safety principles are readily available.

My response: Similarities between aviation and patient care, particularly surgery or other invasive procedures, are readily apparent, but the vast differences between the two are rarely spoken of. Thank goodness for their promise of an open debate because it is long past time when the medical advocates of aviation safety measures in healthcare are forced to recognize both the similarities and the vast differences. I can speak to both.

The authors recognize that when questionable patient care occurs, as it inevitably will, there is typically an unfortunate tendency to turn to the "name/blame/shame cycle", while the quality of healthcare experts prefer to focus on "systems errors".

My response: I struggle with a response to this misguided comment. Patient safety IS NOT an assumed system property! As the second surgeon left to repair the surgical mutilation of patients by their original surgeons I know all too well the dark side of medical care. Revisit my brief conversation with Dr. Wachter in my Introduction: IW: "Dr. Wachter, you speak of systems errors and in my two books I speak of individual practitioner errors. If we brought the two together we would really have something." This name/ blame/ shame nonsense should be considered a slap in the face of any person who, themselves or a loved one has been negligently harmed by a physician. It happens every day somewhere in America! If Sully and his cohorts want the public to wake up and get involved, they need to get involved regarding both systems' errors and individual practitioner errors. (Dr. Wachter said he would "keep me in mind" in 2010. I haven't heard from him.)

The authors have found that, for them at least, "ground zero" for improving healthcare can be found in the hospital board rooms containing the trustees and administrators, and *not at the bedside.*

My response: This statement speaks volumes regarding why the quality of healthcare and patient safety are no better today than over twenty years ago. Neither a hospital board of trustees or any members of our fifty state governments have ever understood that the "buck stops" with the hospital boards, and most hospital board members have never had a clue! This issue is prime material for their promised debate.

The authors have embrace the 4Cs by acknowledging the crisis, joining the cause to make things better, then defining the challenge, and finally taking charge of the efforts for creating the necessary change.

My response: I believe the nation has been aware of the *crisis* for decades, with no sign of improvement. We have long had an army of quality of healthcare experts working diligently to "make healthcare safer, while those same quality of healthcare experts have been "defining the challenge" for over twenty years. And please explain how individual members of the public can "take personal charge"? Too many people, all well meaning, have been trying to incrementally "change a system" that is a non-system, and they don't see that because neither they, or anyone else, has ever attempted to describe it.

The authors recognize the critical need to think innovatively and to act quickly.

My response: Innovative thinking would allow me to offer my checklist system for medical peer review and also allow me to present my three-phase plan on how any state can completely reorganize their state's healthcare delivery system. This should be more material for the promised debate.

Dr. Denham enumerates that integrity, compassion, *accountability*, reliability, and entrepreneurship are the core values of the Texas Medical Institute of Technology of which he is Chairman.

My response: Accountability is an easy word to use, but meaningful accountability at any level of our current healthcare system is difficult, if not impossible to demonstrate. Perhaps Dr. Denham could walk us through the accountability process within the Texas healthcare delivery system.

Sully Sullenberger recognized that the current healthcare status quo has failed and needs to be rejected, while he wishes we were less patient in making changes in how that system is designed so that we might begin to finally reduce the number of needless hospital deaths.

My response: Who has been patient? Brennan and Leape, et al., estimated the annual needless hospital death rate to be 98,000 in 1990! *To Err Is Human* issued a promise to reduce that number by 50 percent in five years. Current estimate of needless hospital deaths, by your count, is 200,000 annually. That is the quality of healthcare experts' status quo, and they are the ones who have failed us.

Dennis Quaid has apparently become sufficiently knowledgeable about healthcare to proclaim that the problem(s) are not due to bad people, but rather to bad systems.

My response: This may come as a surprise to Dennis Quaid, but there are some really bad doctors out there. I suggest he Google: Redding, California. A cardiologist and a cardiovascular surgeon negligently harmed an untold number of patients for years, while members of the administration and medical staff was fully aware and did nothing about it. Until our healthcare system can adequately identify the few, but very significant number of doctors who are not qualified to retain a medical license, there will always be a healthcare safety issue in every state.

The authors recognize Dr. Lucian Leape and particularly Dr. Leape's "frame-changing" 1994 article, 'Error in Medicine' as the initial reference to the need for healthcare to learn from and copy safety measures found in aviation.

My response: He and all others who talk about how to truly make that transition have never understood the similarities and the vast differences in the two endeavors. I am qualified to discuss Gawande's, and Pronovost's checklists and my checklist for individual practitioner peer review.

The authors continue to illustrate how airline pilots take proficiency examinations on a regular basis and within a rigorously controlled system that, unfortunately, is not without its flaws, while they christen Dr. Leape as the Father of patient safety.

My response: Wouldn't the American public love it if their surgeons were forced to take proficiency examinations every six months? I only hope Dr. Leape is invited to participate in the promised debate in order to describe how two decades after his 1990 estimate of 98,000 needless hospital deaths annually and his 1994 article the needless hospital death rate annually has more than doubled.

The authors' major claim to progress being made in patient safety by the use of aviation methods can be attributed to the use of the (WHO) Gawande surgical checklist.

My response: Perhaps Dr. Denham could take several interested people on a tour of rural hospitals in an attempt to determine how well those checklists are being used throughout Texas. South Carolina partnered with Dr. Gawande and his checklist in 2011, but there is no way to determine how consistently that checklist is being utilized in operating rooms in that state.

The authors proclaim that there is always typically more than one root cause of an accident in both aviation and healthcare.

My response: That statement is patently untrue! I lost a roommate and close friend, plus three other crew members to foolish pilot error in South Korea in September 1954, and I have had to provide corrective surgery due to negligence on the part of a first surgeon more than once. Statements such as this diminish the credibility of those seeking to make our healthcare system safer.

The authors are "shocked" that a safety reporting system like the one created for aviation in 1975 has never been created within our healthcare system.

My response: Read this book! States are responsible for our healthcare delivery system, and no state governor or state legislature has ever had a clue regarding their responsibility to create and administer a functional system. Consumers have tolerated this miscarriage because none of the army of quality of healthcare experts, including every school of public health has ever recognized that state responsibility.

The authors, like too many others, are able to recognize that our annual rate of needless hospital deaths is equal to twenty Boeing 747 airliners going down each week.

My response: The reason twice as many patients are needlessly dying in our nation's hospitals now than twenty years ago is because no one has been asking hard questions and demanding full answers from the quality of healthcare experts who control that system. I hope Sully and his cohorts will redirect the focus toward, "Why Have We Not Gotten Further?" (2009)

The authors, rather strangely in my opinion, consider it will be a *great benefit* that their concept of a healthcare NTSB would NOT be required to analyze every healthcare accident in order to make patient safety far better.

My response: Wonderful! But what do you say to the loved ones of a patient who has needlessly died due to the negligent care provided by a physician? That does happen, in probably every hospital in the nation sooner or later. So the authors are O.K. with the current fact that hospitals are the only place in America where an accidental death receives NO immediate review by a source of authority.

The authors do recognize the fact that it has been almost two decades since Dr. Leape wrote his insightful article citing the need for healthcare to learn safety measures form aviation, and they unanimously agree that it is time to do exactly that.

My response: You, we, they, still haven't learned. Aviation safety measures were created and established, both militarily and commercially, in a system with an organizational structure containing clearly defined points of authority and delegated authority. Such absolute necessities have never been present in our nation's healthcare delivery system.

The authors proudly proclaim their unified desire for an "Open Debate"!

My response: YES!! Let's do it! I wanted to debate quality of healthcare experts ever since I wrote *First, Do No Harm* in 2004. Dr. Donald Palmisano, then AMA president, said on an AMA video that this nation needed a healthcare debate. I wrote him requesting such a debate, and he replied that he didn't have time. I flew to Chicago in June 2004 for the AMA annual convention and he and I spoke briefly face to face. There still has been no debate. I am more prepared than ever.

Furthermore, the authors desire a civil debate, focused on real solutions, and authentic governing (whatever that is).

My response: That is what we really need to talk about: solutions. I have a logical and doable three-phase solution that would go far beyond anyone's imagination. I am just looking for audiences of people who want to talk about how to really change healthcare.

The authors claim their desire to become partisan for patients and intend to use every effective political and governmental tool possible in order to reach their goal.

My response: I became *partisan for my patients* over thirty years ago when I testified as the second surgeon in the city in which I practiced. Look what that got me: ostracized. If you truly want to be partisan for patients then find a method of questionable patient care review that will be equally fair to both doctor and patient. I can provide such a peer review system.

In closing their article, the authors claimed that *bureaucracy* is the best device known to man that can turn entrepreneurial energy and financial resources into solid waste, while at the same time their article is predicated on a great need to create another new, enormous *bureaucracy*. However, with no detail, they suggest that their new patient safety creation might be accomplished privately.

My response: I can provide a vastly different solution in your promised debate. The question is, will such a debate ever take place?

I hope this rather elaborate exercise on my part will lead some readers to obtain and read this fascinating collaboration focused on making healthcare far safer in the future. I was so taken by the article that I had obtained by a second source that I sent the following email to Dr. Denham on December 26, 2012.

> Gentlemen,
>
> I was delighted to see in your article, "An NTSB for Healthcare, Learning from Innovation," that you all embrace the need for "civil debate, real solutions, and authentic governing." I hope your season for open debate is still open, because I request an opportunity to debate you regarding the need, prospects, and anticipated benefit of such a new healthcare bureaucracy.
>
> I can provide strong counterpoints to such an enormous undertaking even being considered, and not just based upon our nation's current fiscal difficulties. A healthcare type NTSB would confront many similar obstacles that have always doomed past attempts to create special medical malpractice courts to failure dating back to the mid-seventies. I have considerable experience and understanding regarding special medical malpractice courts and a comparison of the two theoretical processes would be informative, particularly in an open debate.
>
> Plus, I have a better idea. I can provide a detailed plan for the complete reorganization of our nation's healthcare delivery system that is far more logical and doable than a healthcare- type NTSB. Furthermore, my plan would include review of questionable patient care at the site of delivery, rapidly, and within the hospital medical staff.

Debate is defined as a discussion involving opposing viewpoints, and recognizing the national statue of each of you, I assume your declaration that "It is time for civil debate" was made in all sincerity.

I look forward to your response to my request to join you in civil debate regarding such an important national need.

With the utmost courtesy and respect,

Dr. Ira Williams

~

Sully and his cohorts, and particularly Dr. Denham, should first identify who they consider *qualified* and *worthy* to join them in an open debate regarding their proposal. I know I am qualified for such a debate, but I am not optimistic that I would be deemed worthy to share a stage with them.

Periodically, high-ranking individuals in organized medicine and the quality of healthcare field of expertise will publicly acknowledge the *need* for an open debate, but never find a convenient time, or a suitable site, or more likely, an opponent sufficiently worthy to discuss opposing viewpoints. I certainly agree with them that the nation could derive great benefit from such a debate. I hope that the American public will view their invitation for an open debate to be a test for their individual and collective sincerity.

I apologize if my responses have been too severe, but as stated in their article, too many people have been needlessly dying in our nation's hospitals for far too long. I am passionate in wanting to contribute to making our healthcare delivery system far better. I know how to do that! I am seeking an opportunity to contribute to helping make healthcare in America far safer.

This is why I am well qualified to offer a rational counterpoint to their quest for a new federal bureaucracy, and why I believe the efforts to create a Healthcare National Safety Board will be a huge waste of time and money, and ultimately end in a similar manner to special medical malpractice courts.

Special Medical Malpractice Courts

Special medical malpractice courts were a theoretical attempt to better control the constantly growing medical malpractice litigation crisis. I have particularly deep understanding of the four-decade, multiple attempts to create such courts and why each of those attempts ended in abject failure, and why the multiple, unsuccessful attempts to create special medical malpractice courts provide a reliable indication of why the quest for a healthcare clone of the NTSB will suffer a similar fate.

But first one must understand what initiated such a prolong search for a solution to a national dilemma. The Medical Malpractice Crisis hit every practicing physician and dentist without warning, like the first wave of a tsunami in the mid-1970s, and turned the private practice of medicine and dentistry upside down. Some insurance companies stopped writing malpractice insurance all together and others changed how those policies were written, while also increasing their premiums significantly. I know because I was one of those practitioners, along with my partners, who were left to wonder, "What just happened?" We were completely blindsided.

The private practice of medicine and dentistry has never been the same since; and like tsunamis, the Medical Malpractice Crisis also continued to send additional waves of malpractice litigation crisis every succeeding decade. Plus that crisis remains just as perplexing and just as unresolved today as it was in the mid-seventies.

Back to special medical malpractice courts and the continuing efforts to make a theoretical solution become a functional reality . . . .

Wisconsin Special Medical Malpractice Courts

Never let a serious crisis go to waste! The Wisconsin governor and legislature of that time did not. Someone, source or sources unknown to me, suggested that special medical malpractice courts were just what the doctor(s) ordered. Thus a two-tier system of such courts was created, and I know most people will find that the basis of those two tiers will titillate the reader, but such was the economic times of the mid-seventies.

IF a patient (plaintiff) sued a doctor for 10,000 dollars or less, the special court would be comprised of one attorney (judge), one doctor, and one layperson.

IF the claim were for over that 10,000-dollar threshold, the special court would be comprised of one attorney (judge), two doctors, and two lay-people. These special courts would conduct their affairs in all ways similar to civil court proceedings, including the discovery process, depositions, and such.

Wisconsin's system of special medical malpractice courts gained legislative life about the time I was becoming ensnared into the dilemma of being the second surgeon requested to treat the results of a patient's current condition caused by the clearly negligent care from their original surgeon or surgeons.

Dilemma is the proper word to describe the unholy predicament the second surgeon will always find themselves in when faced with trying to make the best of a very bad situation for the patient, while being forced to confront the professional and ethical obligations that second surgeon has to his new patient, his colleague, his community, his profession, and himself. Such a dilemma occurs in our nation's healthcare system all too often, and is truly a no-win situation. Unfortunately, in almost all such cases, the second surgeon refuses to participate in any type of review of the first surgeon's surgical performance and expertise.

It had never crossed my mind that someday I might be called upon to judge the patient care of another surgeon. When ultimately faced with that prospect, I was sorely conflicted. Only a fool breaks the code of silence, particularly in their own community, and that is why there is rare evidence of such "fools" in any medical community in America. I felt I had to answer questions for those who had a right to ask me questions about those patient's conditions as I found them, what standard of care had they been provided by the first surgeon(s), and details of what forms of treatment were required for me to treat their postoperative condition, and attempt to establish an acceptable result. That professional obligation I felt, in time, would cost me my ability to continue to practice oral and maxillofacial surgery in Madison, Wisconsin, but it would ultimately lead me to write this, my third book on our healthcare delivery system.

I was called to testify before two tier-two special medical malpractice courts. The first case involved a simple fracture of the lower jaw of a middle-aged woman. IF treated properly, she would have spent one or two nights in the hospital after one brief surgical procedure in the operating room, and would have been fully healed in about six weeks. Such was not the case in her sad story.

The second case involved a middle-aged retarded male with a functional IQ of a five- to six-year-old who had been "surgically mutilated" (my court- room description) over a period of five months, including five surgical procedures. In both cases the two surgeons in the first case, and the surgeon in the second case, had broken every rule of an acceptable standard of care for their respective patients; and in each court proceeding, the surgeons were found guilty of medical malpractice. The second surgeon (older brother) in the first case was made chief of Surgery at his hospital the next year after that simple fracture debacle, and in the same year both brothers handled a similar case of simple lower jaw fracture even more poorly.

Wisconsin Special Medical Malpractice Courts can be summarized in these two conclusions: They were a judicial disgrace and after about ten years of such disgrace, the governor and state legislature killed their theoretical cure for medical malpractice. But unfortunately, theoretical solutions for major national problems have a propensity to resurface.

AMA Medical Liability Project

The AMA-Specialty Society Medical Liability Project (later named the AMA Medical Liability Project) was being birthed about the time Wisconsin was burying their judicial deformity. This was described in the *Chicago Sun Times* on January 17, 1988 in an article called "Lifting the burden of malpractice: Take it out of the courts.

Basically the AMA system would adjudicate medical malpractice claims by an administrative agency, either a modified state medical licensing board or a brand-new state agency. Also, in the pre-hearing stage, all claims would be quickly reviewed, *and those with merit* would be submitted to an appropriate expert (sources of such expertise to be determined later).

This entire project had been in development for almost two years before its 1988 unveiling and was being seriously evaluated for implementation by medical societies in two states, Utah and Vermont. There was one major fly in this new AMA ointment: Federal funding for the testing of this model in those two states would be necessary, but fortunately for all, it was not forthcoming.

Medical Malpractice Solutions, co-edited by four physicians and attorneys and published in 1989, devoted one entire chapter in their book to this particular "malpractice solution" as one of the potential solutions. Open with a bang and close without a whimper can best describe the legacy of the AMA Medical Liability Project. I could find no one at AMA headquarters in Chicago who had ever even heard of that effort when I was researching their Liability Project for *First, Do No Harm* in 2003. So far, none of the Medical Malpractice Solutions promised in that rather large book of the same name, or by its dozen or so experts, has yet to take effect and solve our ongoing medical malpractice dilemma.

But special medical malpractice courts and theoretical solutions for our ever-present medical malpractice crisis apparently refuse to die.

Newt Gingrich and Common Good

Newt Gingrich and "never let a major crisis go to waste" are a match made in heaven. Newt, with some initial help from New York attorney Philip Howard, made a lot of money while beating the drum for special medical malpractice courts. Their fruitful collaboration for both appears to have followed this timeline.

Congressman Gingrich returned to private life in 1999 and began to create multiple businesses and nonprofit ventures. Attorney Howard wrote *The Collapse of the Common Good, How America's Lawsuit Culture Undermines Our Freedom* in 2001. Thus, in 2002, was born: Common Good.

Common Good

Anyone tempted to fall in love with the prospect of a healthcare clone of the NTSB *should be forced* to first study, in detail, the history of Common Good. The following is a brief memoir of information taken from their literature and my experiences meeting some of their staff over several years and attending two of their widely advertised public forums. Common Good is a nonpartisan, nonprofit organization founded in 2002 with the mission of rebuilding reliable legal structure that will permit Americans to use their common sense. Providence greatly assisted their startup by uniting Attorney Howard with Newt Gingrich as demonstrated by a colorful six-page, seven-by-ten brochure entitled "An Urgent Call for Special Health Courts." Headlines in its inner pages included:

Unreliable Justice Is Destroying American Healthcare, How Special Health Courts Would Solve the Problem, How Special Health Courts Would Work, Coming Together for Our Common Good, and two facing pages:

These Leaders Agree, the Time Has Come for Special Health Courts.

Included in that list of almost 100 leaders were numerous university and medical school presidents, former US senators, a former and a future US attorney general, and leaders throughout our healthcare delivery system, plus, of course, Mr. Howard and Hon. Newt Gingrich.

During a promotional trip to NYC in July 2004 for my book, *First, Do No Harm*, I visited the very small Common Good office and met with what appeared to be their only staff person in that office, a delightful young lady who would probably prefer not to be named. I did leave a signed copy of my book for Attorney Howard and later wrote him a letter expressing interest in their efforts and my desire to share insight. I received no response.

Common Good's primary point of action was (where else?) in their Washington DC office. I visited that office on a couple of occasions while in DC and met with Paul J. Barringer III, general counsel and director of Operations. The last time Paul and I spoke, my parting remark was, "Paul, we seek the same goal, but choose to take a different path. Perhaps someday we will be able to join forces."

I attended the Public Forum: Common Good and the Harvard School of Public Health called "Health Courts and Administrative Compensation: Opportunities For Safety Enhancement" on November 8, 2006.

The half-day event included three separate presentations and two panel discussions before an audience I estimated to be approximately 100. It was funded by the Robert Wood Johnson Foundation. A small contingent representing the Wyoming Healthcare Commission showed particular interest in this form of medical malpractice regulation. I made no attempt to contribute to the discussions, but left that gathering conflicted between what I knew about the real world of trying to judge the questionable patient care of another practitioner and all that I felt that had never been mentioned or even recognized by any other person present, presenter, or attendee.

"Towards a More Reliable System of Medical Justice: Opportunities, Challenges and Lessons Learned" was scheduled for November 18, 2008, and again funded by Robert Wood Johnson Foundation. I planned to attend, but wanted to speak to someone in their office prior to that event. Jenny Foreit had replaced Paul Barringer as general counsel, although Paul was still scheduled to participate in the proceedings, and in fact did. Jenny was kind enough to speak with me by phone a couple of weeks prior to the event, and I believe our brief, cordial conversation goes right to the heart of why special medical malpractice courts AND a healthcare clone of the NTSB are both theoretical considerations that can never become reality—and should never be pursued.

I began our conversation with a brief description of South Carolina, i.e., moderate in size and population, having three metropolitan communities, sixty-five acute care hospitals and sixty-eight surgery centers. I then asked Jenny two questions:

> **IW:** Special malpractice courts require two individuals with specific expertise. Without naming names of course, how many individuals of each type can Common Good identify at this time?

JENNY: None.

IW: How many special courts would South Carolina, or any other state of similar size need?

JENNY: We don't know.

I did attend that meeting and did not raise either question at any time in the proceeding. They knew what points they were seeking to pursue, and I knew my perspective would not fit into their well-established path toward a more reliable system of medical justice. Personally, I have always believed they have been looking at a way to confront medical malpractice through the wrong end of their telescope.

It appears that, as of 2012, the Robert Wood Johnson Foundation has greatly reduced or stopped entirely its funding of Common Good. Common Good web site shows an office now in Brooklyn, New York. I can only judge that the time, effort, and money expended upon this quest, based upon wishful thinking, to have been a colossal failure; and if any good can come out of it that will hopefully be for those seeking a healthcare clone of NTSB to consider the similarities in their efforts.

Newt Gingrich became so enamored with the prospects of special medical malpractice courts, and other healthcare issues in which he possessed no real expertise that he created his Center for Health Transformation. I made several attempts to connect with his staff in his Center for Health Transformation Atlanta office, but to no avail.

Wall Street Journal reported in April 2012—Georgia: "Ex-Gingrich Think Tank Files for Bankruptcy: A healthcare think tank started by Newt Gingrich has filed for Chapter 7 bankruptcy, according to federal court filings, closing the most profitable of Mr. Gingrich's former enterprises and potentially putting a big piece of his net worth in jeopardy."

Summary: After ten years of concentrated effort to build a case for how special medical malpractice courts could somehow miraculously solve our dilemma of medical malpractice there is still nothing of substance to support such effort. The healthcare delivery system would be better off if someone had the ability to perform euthanasia on this entire judicial deformity. Four decades of failure should be enough.

Greater Summary: Wisconsin, AMA Medical Liability Project, and Common Good: How long must it take for people to understand that special medical malpractice courts started out to be some person's or persons' dream and became a quality of healthcare nightmare. Healthcare NTSB worshipers, be careful what you pray for.

Side note: At the end of that November 18, 2008, Common Good event in DC, I spoke with one of the presenters whose bio listed him as a health policy analyst best known for crafting a new progressive agenda for healthcare. I told him I was in the process of writing my second book on healthcare, and I would be offering a rudimentary diagram of the organizational structure of our current healthcare system plus some suggestions on how to begin to reorganize it. He requested that I send him an email with three to five bullet points describing my book, and that IF I couldn't describe my book in three to five points, then I probably didn't really understand the subject.

His was not the first or the last time I had been asked to describe my book in three to five brief points, and I consider such requests to be insults! Not to me! (I'm not important. I am just the messenger, and throughout history there has been a very unfortunate tendency to "kill the messenger.") Such a request insults the subject—our healthcare system! YOURS AND MINE. That system directly impacts every living person, plus those yet unborn. It is almost 20 percent of our entire national economy, and it is SICK! Those who think a thumbnail description of what ails healthcare should be sufficient best be willing to continue to keep what we have now. There are too many pseudo-experts like Newt Gingrich and Philip Howard who think they understand our healthcare problems; but unfortunately, they don't.

Sully and I Share a Common Bond

Sully and I share a similar misgiving regarding our past military life. We were both trained in combat aircraft, but fortunately never faced an enemy. Naturally, we are both left to wonder, "Would I have performed the way I like to think I would have performed?" There can never be a definitive answer, but we are each left to wonder.

On Saturday, October 28, 1962, I was awakened at midnight and told to report to our unit at the military ramp at Memphis Municipal Airport at 8:00 a.m. I was back on active duty thanks to the Cuban Crisis. That event reduced my internship from twelve months to ten, and appeared to end my process of seeking acceptance to an oral surgery residency program. Our Air Force Reserve Troop Carrier unit had focused most of our training on dropping Army parachute trainees at Fort Benning, Georgia; Fort Bragg, North Carolina; and Fort Campbell, Kentucky.

If we had invaded Cuba, things would have been quite different for our unit. We would have been the "first boots on the ground," and I do mean we. We would have assault landed at the missile sites and let the troops out the back ramp. That would have instantly turned me into an untrained infantry officer with only a .45 on my hip. Having spent most of my time in my internship in oral surgery with a dental surgeon who spent time in World War II Europe in a MASH unit, I knew that once on the ground I would need to be able to utilize my surgical expertise, such as it was at that time. I bought a Boy Scout backpack and created an emergency kit so that I could extract teeth as needed, close wounds, and wire jaws together. I could certainly do far more good with that kit than I ever could have with that .45. I kept that backpack for quite a few years, just as a reminder of how a turn of events can redirect one's life.

I was selected for the crew to represent our unit at Homestead Air Force Base, south of Miami, the week after that crisis ceased to be a crisis. President Kennedy had hoped to honor those units recalled to active duty, but his schedule did not permit that ceremony. After five days of staying close to the phone, we were told to return home. Our, and similar units, were awarded the Presidential Unit Citation. Air Force Major Rudolph Anderson, a U-2 pilot from Greenville, South Carolina, was the only combat fatality during the Cuban Crisis. His memorial was rededicated in Greenville in October 2012.

During my three-year oral and maxillofacial surgery residency at Marquette University and the VA Hospital in Milwaukee, Wisconsin, I was also a member of the Wisconsin Air National Guard unit as a navigator. That unit's mission was air-to-air refueling, but it also had its own aero club. That provided me with the opportunity to obtain my private pilot license (single engine). This led me to another great flying thrill. I was able to arrange a training mission to Frankfurt, Germany, in late June 1965 that just coincidentally matched the schedule for the Second International Association of Oral and Maxillofacial Surgeons Conference in Copenhagen, Denmark.

I had to have been the only American oral surgery resident at that conference, but a greater thrill awaited me at the airport. My crew landed at Copenhagen to pick me up. While the flight plan was being filed and the plane refueled, I noticed some of our crew across the runway gathered around where a Danish Air Force glider was taking off and landing. I hurried over and got in line. When it became my turn, I mentioned that I was a pilot. The Danish lieutenant said, "Get in front." It can't get much better than flying a glider over Copenhagen, Denmark, on a gorgeous summer day. The pilot never touched the controls, and I nailed the landing.

While Sully and I never experienced combat, people need to understand that flying training missions in combat aircraft is not like a walk in the park. I lost that new, but close friend, along with three other crew members in that crash in the mountains of Japan in the fall of 1954. During our island-hopping return from Japan to our new base in Florida, we had made our last overnight refueling stop at Tinker Air Force Base Oklahoma City, Oklahoma. Our flight of four planes were sitting near the active runway, awaiting takeoff instructions, as a flight of single-engine fighters began to land in sequence. Unfortunately, one of the pilots failed to nail his landing, and attempted to go around. At the far end of the runway, and having failed to gain altitude or sufficient airspeed for control, a wingtip caught the ground and he exploded like a napalm bomb. The active runway was closed for some time; but after approximately an hour, our flight of four was cleared for takeoff. As we cleared the runway, every crew member in those four planes was drawn to look to our left—and all we could see was how that plane and that pilot had become a large patch of white ash.

I have lost friends and attended too many military funerals, and participated in folding the flag after the highly emotional twenty-one- gun salute and the missing man flyover too many times. One does not have to experience combat in order to understand the cost of becoming combat ready.

Old soldiers can go on and on, but I hope I have made my case that I am fully qualified to participate in any discussions regarding how to incorporate aviation safety procedures into the efforts to make our healthcare delivery system far better. I can hardly wait for that debate. I just hope it will truly be an open and courteous sharing of qualified viewpoints, focused on issues and not persons, and with only positive intent.

But who's been missing thus far in the concerted efforts to make healthcare far safer? AMA and state medical examining boards, except for the AMA efforts through their self-centered National Patient Safety Foundation. Now for a look into the real AMA as so many people, both inside and outside the medical profession, know them to be.

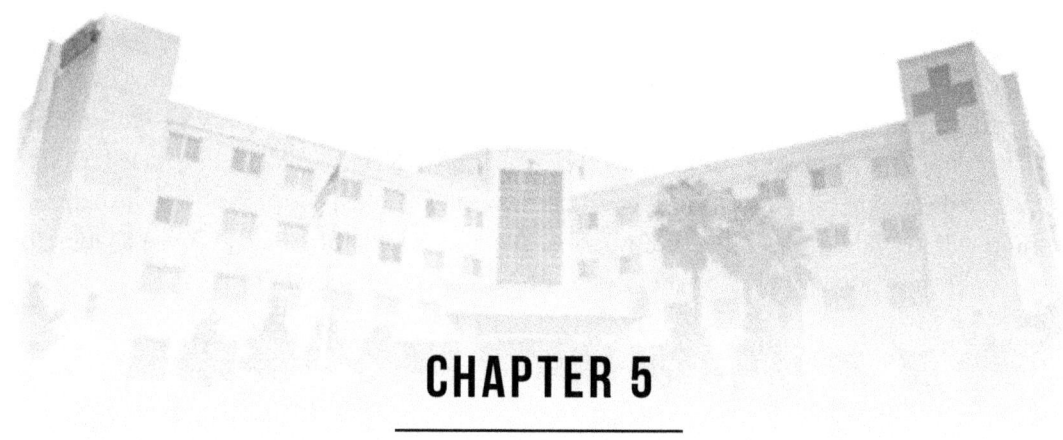

CHAPTER 5

BEHIND THE AMA CURTAIN

AMA Corruption of Malpractice Litigation

I love the medical and dental professions and my oral surgery specialty, and have long hoped to be considered one of the best friends the medical profession has ever had. However, if that old saying, "The truth will set you free!" is accurate, then this chapter might help to set free our medical profession from a long history of putting personal interests first before the best interests of patients.

Without a doubt, this book demonstrates, in the "experts" own words, how the leadership of our medical profession, in every state, has collaborated to *corrupt* the entire system of medical malpractice litigation (Sue or forget it). I accept full responsibility for sharing the information I have openly obtained.

A chronological path of parallel events, one involving a highly questionable hospital death and the other involving the highest level of leaders within the AMA and every state's medical societies, must be followed in order to take a reader behind the curtain of how organized medicine seeks to deny the public legal justice. Try to imagine your reaction if a similar set of circumstances occurred in your life. For some, the events described here will become all too real. Others have already found out about such things the hard way.

First Event

1975: A young North Carolina couple celebrated the joyful birth of a son. Unfortunately, their initial joy was tempered when their infant was diagnosed with congenital hydrocephalus, the swelling of the brain due to excess buildup of cerebrospinal fluid. There are certain factors regarding cerebral hydrocephalus that must be understood before proceeding with the important aspects of this first event.

Congenital hydrocephalus requires a neurosurgeon to insert a cerebral shunt (a one-way pump/drain), between the brain cavity and other areas within the patient's body in order to redirect the excess cerebrospinal fluid (CSF). The common symptoms of intracranial pressure from the buildup of CSF from hydrocephalus include headache, nausea, vomiting, vision problems, and lethargy. If the buildup of CSF is untreated, brain damage and death can result.

Note: Once the initial shunt is placed, it will likely need to be replaced periodically. Furthermore, this type of surgical procedure, like any other surgical procedure, is susceptible to a number of complications, even possibly leading to death, but many people can live healthy lives IF provided with adequate medical care. Each of those points plays an important part in this first event.

1995: Bill, the central figure in this first event, had successfully dealt with his congenital abnormality for almost twenty years, including periodic shunt replacement procedures, sufficient to allow him to leave home and attend an in-state university. During his academic year, Bill faced the need for another shunt replacement procedure. Bill consulted with neurosurgeon #1 and the replacement procedure was agreed upon and scheduled. Bill was also told, and accepted, that following that procedure Bill's postoperative care would be the responsibility of the surgeon on call, neurosurgeon #2. The surgery appeared to go well; but about four hours later, and after neurosurgeon #2 had assumed responsibility for neurosurgeon #1's patients, Bill got a headache and grew agitated. There appeared to be some indication that the nursing staff called neurosurgeon #2 to report Bill's complaint of increasing headache, but neurosurgeon #2 did not immediately respond by coming to see his new patient (medical responsibility).

The rest of Bill's unfortunate story can be summarized with these few details: by the time neurosurgeon #2 arrived at Bill's bedside, his patient (Bill) was in critical condition; he had stopped breathing. Bill was revived, and neurosurgeon #2 performed emergency brain surgery. But that surgery proved to be too late. Bill was put on a respirator and died eighteen days later. Bill's parents were left to grieve the perhaps needless, but certainly highly questionable, loss of their son. They were also left with the option: "Sue or Forget It".

Sue or Forget It

Throughout the history of healthcare in America, the public has overwhelmingly been left with medical malpractice litigation as the primary source for the review of questionable patient care. Bill's parents found themselves on the horns of that dilemma while trying to cope with having to bury their young son, and wondering what happened. Bill's parents decided they must enter that strange and adversarial land of medical malpractice litigation, where each side is so often determined to "take no prisoners!"

What do people need to know if and when they feel they must sue a doctor?
    First, they must understand that they must deal with:

- The psychological burden of instantly being seen as a *pariah* within their medical community (there will be definite repercussions).
- Endurance, because malpractice litigation typically requires three or more years, and the stigma is constant.
- Financial burden, even with a contingency basis. (I never served as an expert witness for financially sound plaintiffs, but I only served as an expert witness for those plaintiffs who I sincerely believed deserved their day in court.)

Second, certain absolutes are needed to initiate the litigation process:
- An attorney qualified in medical malpractice litigation. (I had the misfortune to be involved in a malpractice trial with a good attorney who was, unfortunately, lacking in medical malpractice litigation experience. That trial did not go well.)
- Qualified expert witnesses (a vanishing breed), because *there is NO medical malpractice without expert witness testimony.*
- *Res ipsa loquitur* (Latin: the thing speaks for itself). No expert witness is required IF they amputate the wrong limb, etc. This exception is a malpractice litigation rarity, requested more often by plaintiffs' attorneys than allowed by trial judges.

The Die is Cast

1997: Bill's parents made the determination that they needed to enter the medical malpractice litigation arena, and they were able to fulfill the first requirement. They obtained qualified medical malpractice attorneys. Those attorneys were able to acquire the services of a Florida-based neurosurgeon, experienced as an expert witness in such cases, and who just happened to have a North Carolina medical license (not that that was necessary, but that fact becomes important to the rest of this story).

Note: I obtained a Wisconsin license to practice oral surgery at the completion of my three-year residency in Milwaukee that allowed me to practice oral surgery in Madison, Wisconsin. I also possessed a license to practice in Tennessee, my home state, obtained in 1961, and another license to practice in Louisiana obtained in the summer of 1962 during my internship. I retained both as active licenses for many years.

Medical malpractice litigation process requires several preliminary steps:
- Qualified attorney to obtain all medical records, review those records and accept the plaintiffs as clients, and obtain an expert witness to do the same.
- Expert witnesses must review the records, determine if he or she is qualified to testify and if the records support an expert witness opinion that the patient care did not meet a reasonable standard of care, then accept the responsibility as an expert witness in that case.
- Judge must determine that all necessary requirements have been satisfied in order to set the case for trial. Some states require expert witnesses to first certify in writing

the factors upon which they will based their testimony of substandard care. I have provided several such letters for judicial acceptance and was never turned down.
- Discovery process begins following judicial approval of the plaintiff's case. Depositions are taken from defendant doctors, plaintiffs, expert witnesses, and any other persons, as determined by the trial judge. Expert witness depositions are taken under oath, reviewed by the person deposed in order to make corrections, if necessary, and accepted as equal to sworn testimony given in a trial.

1997: The neurosurgeon expert witness provided his deposition in the plaintiffs' (Bill's parents) malpractice cases against neurosurgeons #1 and #2 and the hospital for the negligent death of their son. Neurosurgeon #1 and the hospital settled their cases with the plaintiffs. [Note: I have given about forty malpractice depositions in surgical malpractice cases involving both physicians and oral surgeons. Far more of those cases settled after my deposition than later went to trial.]

One might assume that this sad saga of the highly questionable death of a young man would be nearing its end, but the full details of Bill's death would not be known for another nine years, and with further long-standing ramifications in the world of medical malpractice litigation and the AMA/50 state medical societies collaborative Litigation Center.

Two separate events, Bill's death in North Carolina and the creation of the Litigation Center, coincidentally came together over a five year period and enabled the AMA to clearly demonstrate who comes first in their professional obligations: doctors or patients and their grieving loved ones.

First event: Bill's parents, for reasons of their own, but understandable to me, elected not to pursue further litigation efforts against neurosurgeon #2 that would require them to relive Bill's questionable death in a trial months away, and before a jury of people with no medical expertise. Therefore, the only questions ever asked and answered regarding the circumstances of Bill's untimely death were contained in that expert witness deposition (the key to further events during the next nine years); and they were presumably asked and answered.

Five years later, the AMA and the North Carolina Medical Society decided that the malpractice litigation review of Bill's highly questionable death DID NOT meet "their standards of medical review."

Second event (also in 1997): AMA began formulating a process to unite themselves with all fifty state medical societies in the creation of what became the Litigation Center about the same time as Bill's highly questionable death and the malpractice litigation process was seemingly coming to a close.

Bill's death and malpractice litigation process became the centerpiece used to christen that new AMA/state medical societies creation to protect doctors from "evil" plaintiffs' expert witnesses, who just happen to be an absolute necessity in almost every medical malpractice civil trial ever conducted in our courts for over 150 years.

Testifying is Practicing Medicine

AMA policy says that when a physician gives medical legal testimony, it's considered the practice of medicine and it should be subject to peer review. The Association's House of Delegates passed the resolution in 1997 and reaffirmed it in 1998, 1999, and 2000.

1997 – The Beginning

1997: Bill's parents accepted the settlement with neurosurgeon #1 and the hospital, and decided not to further pursue litigation against neurosurgeon #2, even though he was the surgeon on call who failed to respond immediately to Bill's clinical sign of possible postoperative complication. Simultaneously, the AMA House of Delegates was laying the groundwork for future assaults on patient's expert witnesses.

Before moving on to the second event, and the events to follow, there are several considerations to be aware of regarding the AMA, and all associations.

Associations are *membership organizations*. As such, they have NO authority over their members. Certainly, any threat of possible conduct review by an association would be easily met with, "I just resigned my membership." Yet federal and state decision makers have always accepted medical and hospital associations as though they possessed such authority over their members.

AMA is estimated to have less than 30 percent of the nation's doctors as members, yet their House of Delegates presumed they were sufficiently powerful to suddenly (over four years) make new expert witness law, and have that new law accepted throughout organized medicine. And, folks, they did it—and got away with it. Now I will show you how they got away with it.

Litigation Center of the AMA-State Medical Societies

The AMA began creating the Litigation Center and recruiting state medical societies to join them in the late 1990s. They were successful in having all fifty state medical societies as active members by 2003. This tale of two simultaneous events involving the questionable death of Bill in 1995 and the assumed closing of his parent's litigation process in 1997 gained new life thanks to the AMA-State Medical Societies Litigation Center.

Of the Litigation Center's eleven-member Executive Committee, nine of those members represented eight state medical societies and the District of Columbia in 2002. But one Executive Committee member stands out from the rest regarding Bill's questionable death seven years earlier.

Stephen W. Keene was then (and continues to be) North Carolina Medical Society general counsel and deputy executive vice president of Government Affairs and Health Policy.

Second Event Begins—But How?

Who called whom first? Did neurosurgeon #2, still burning with indignation five years after Bill's parents had ended their quest for medical justice, somehow hear about this relatively new AMA-State Medical Society Litigation Center for the *peer review* of expert witness testimony? OR, did NCMS General Counsel Stephen Keene recognize an opportunity to test this new professional device for reviewing any plaintiff's (patient's) expert witness testimony?

As an experienced plaintiff's expert witness in numerous malpractice cases across the nation, I know what I believe about who called whom first, but I will leave it to others to speculate. After being called a "hired gun" by every defense attorney I ever faced, I understand all too well the medical profession's mindset regarding malpractice litigation. But fortunately we have additional information to help in making such a judgment.

Expert witness fighting loss of medical license over testimony: Greenville News, September 2, 2002

I had been familiar with the AMA making expert witness testimony equal to patient care, and their creation of the Litigation Center. But neither I, or anyone else knew how that combination of AMA efforts might be utilized until the first application of these new professional powers became real thanks to the additional might of the North Carolina Medical Board when they agreed to participate. Several newspapers in both Carolinas described the event and the wide range of responses to that event.

Neurosurgeon #2, who had not agreed to settle the malpractice claim brought by Bill's parents, and yet, who was passively released from that claim apparently had continue to "burn with rage" over his assured belief that [Expert Witness] had lied about his actions and responses to Bill's critical condition under oath in his deposition. Furthermore, the AMA Litigation Center, North Carolina Medical Society and the North Carolina Medical Board reassured him that they concurred. [Expert Witness] was deemed, by the above three professional entities, to have been either dishonest or incompetent when he clearly misstated the standard of care in North Carolina (in their collective opinions).

[Expert Witness] had 20 years of experience as an expert witness, but he (and no other expert witness up until then) had never been forced to defend his conduct and testimony to a state medical board before when he was contacted in April 2002 and told the NCMB had scheduled a hearing regarding his testimony in that case in July. His request for a delay in the Board hearing scheduled for July 19, 2002, due to a schedule conflict, was denied by the Board.

The Board found [Expert Witness] had repeatedly made factual assertions without an evidentiary or good faith basis and had misrepresented the applicable standard of care. The Board determined that was unprofessional conduct and revoked his North Carolina license on July 19, 2002. *The Board voted unanimously after twenty minutes of deliberation.*

The Board President, the AMA President, and the executive vice president and chief executive officer of the Federation of State Medical Boards were unanimous in their support of this demonstration of medical profession retribution so necessary to insure that only expert witness testimony of the highest order will be permitted in the future. Others, not so closely aligned with the medical profession saw a much more darker outcome for the future of medical malpractice litigation. Thankfully this story does not end with doctors in North Carolina popping champagne corks.

[Expert Witness] appealed the Board's ruling and the order to revoke his North Carolina medical license (which also threatened the status of his Florida license and his professional future) in April 2003 and the Board's decision to revoke his license was vacated and replaced with a one year suspension in 2004. [Expert Witness] was still not done.

[Expert Witness] appealed that appellate decision in 2004, and the next appellate decision by the same judge made no change in his previous decision. [Expert Witness] appealed that decision in 2005, and the true facts of this entire matter finally were exposed.

North Carolina Court of Appeals Filed: 6 June 2006

Neurosurgeon #2 had recorded in the patient's record that the patient's cerebral spinal fluid was *not under increased pressure at the time of his second surgery.* However the patient did not respond to that second surgery and subsequently died.

[Expert Witness] was accused by defense attorneys using his deposition testimony during the trial that he had accused neurosurgeon #2 of falsifying medical records. [Expert Witness] denied ever claiming such an accusation. However [Expert Witness] had testified that there were four clinically evident reasons for his conclusion that the patient's cerebral spinal fluid pressure had to be elevated. Therefore [Expert Witness] had difficulty believing neurosurgeon #2 notation to the contrary.

It was further pointed out that there were at least three highly qualified healthcare professionals in close proximity to the patient when neurosurgeon #2 removed the original drain that had been placed by neurosurgeon #1. An anesthesiologist, a surgical (scrub) nurse and a circulating nurse were present at that moment and yet in testimony it was stated that nobody else who witnessed the removal of that drain "recalls whether spinal fluid spurted out or not." Basically the only one who commented on that was neurosurgeon #2, and the others participating in that surgical procedure "saw no evil, heard no evil, and certainly, spoke no evil."

The North Carolina Medical Board is statutorily imbued with the authority to regulate the practice of medicine and surgery for the benefit and protection of the people of North Carolina. The board has the power to deny, annul, suspend, or revoke the license of a license holder found by the Board to have committed unprofessional conduct. As such the Board is an occupational licensing agency, which is governed by Article 3A of the North Carolina Administrative Procedure Act. Occupational licensing agency means any board which is established for the primary purpose of regulating the entry of persons into, and/or the conduct of persons with a particular profession, and which is authorized to issue and revoke licenses.

North Carolina Medical Board, in revoking [Expert Witness'] license based that action upon multiple reasons to support their contention that [Expert Witness] had absolutely no direct evidence to support his extremely serious accusation.

The Superior Court ruled that his finding was supported by substantial evidence in the record including the four clinically evident reasons [Expert Witness] stated. These observations provided a good faith evidentiary basis for [Expert Witness'] opinion that neurosurgeons #2 notation was not credible. Furthermore the record is clear that [Expert Witness] was content to state no more than his opinion that neurosurgeon #2 note in the patient's record was faulty.

Superior Court three-judge appellate panel found no evidence in the record to support the Medical Board's decision to revoke [Expert Witness] license. Therefore the Board erred by finding that [Expert Witness] leveled a groundless accusation and that the previous Superior Court appeals processes had erroneously applied the whole record test to affirm the Medical Boards determination. Therefore the Superior Court's previous orders affirming the Board's decision was reversed and the disciplinary proceedings against [Expert Witness] were dismissed. The Court's final order reversed and remanded by unanimous consent of the three judges in June 2006.

North Carolina Medical Board's executive director was quoted in a state newspaper the day after the North Carolina Court of Appeals had revoked that Board's previous finding in 2002, "The Medical Board's position was and probably still is that [Expert Witness] testimony in that case was at best reckless."

Eleven years of professional tragedy compounded by professional malfeasance and every state medical society still has a Litigation Center component, so I will provide some additional summation to compare to the NCMB executive director's unqualified estimation of neurosurgical testimony.

Question never asked: Where was the NCMB, with their profound expertise regarding neurosurgical standards of care, in 1995 when young, otherwise healthy, Bill died under highly questionable immediate post- operative circumstances? No where to be found, and in spite of the above description of their responsibility to the people of their state.

Neurosurgeon #1 received his original license to practice medicine in North Carolina in 1964 and he did not reactivate his license in 1998. Neurosurgeon #2 gained his license in 1993 and the NCMB web site indicates that he continues to practice and teach neurosurgery and has NO medical malpractice charges noted on his record

NCMB also has a very long history of contributing numerous members to leadership positions in the Federation of State Medical Boards, particularly in the last several decades, and during the time period of this entire matter.

Where can [Expert Witness] go to regain his professional reputation? The American public would be well served if someone were to capture the complete details of this two-event saga, beginning with young Bill's highly questionable death and the Frankenstein-like creation of the AMA/ Medical Societies Litigation Center and ending with the North Carolina Court of Appeals unmasking of this entire professional charade in June 2006.

I still have copies of "lies under oath" given in a deposition by a defense expert witness who just happened to be the chairman of a Surgery Department at the local medical school and teaching hospital. I wager the AMA-Medical Societies Litigation Center has never collaborated with a state medical examining board to review the sworn testimony of an expert witness who happened to be testifying in defense of the accused practitioner.

[Remember when I mentioned that hospitals (and surgery centers) are the only places in America where an accidental death receives no immediate review by a state source of authority?]

These parallel events, involving Bill's unfortunate death and the emergence of the new and dynamic AMA-State Medical Societies Litigation Center, aided by very willing state medical boards, raises far more questions and provides far fewer answers than the involved components of organized medicine would wish to confront. But I do raise some of those questions here, and provide some of my highly opinionated responses. I name names and give dates (if and when necessary), because it is impossible to create a well-defined picture of a complex issue unless one connects the dots with the facts. So let's begin with MEDICAL MALPRACTICE.

What is Medical Malpractice and Who decides?

First, I despise the term "medical malpractice." All doctors are human, all humans make mistakes; therefore, even the best doctors make mistakes; and as we have seen, you can take Dr. Atul Gawande's word for that.

"Questionable Patient Care" (is it or isn't it?) is a far better term for two reasons: "medical malpractice" is a pejorative that instantly labels an unknown as an accepted negative; and not all medical complications are due to substandard care. I would always support a doctor in the review of a case where all reasonable patient care had been provided—as I would the patient in cases where substandard care was clearly evident.

Evolution of the Medical Malpractice Dilemma

Doctors don't know how to fairly judge another doctor's questionable patient care, and they never have known or ever attempted to try to learn how. The leadership in our nation's medical profession took the easy way out and left the public with no other option except: "Sue or forget it!" throughout the entire history of their profession.

Organized Medicine (One of its Finest hours)

Organized medicine was represented solely by the founding of the American Medical Association (AMA) in 1847, followed by the American College of Surgeons (ACS) in 1913, and the American College of Physicians (ACP) in 1915. Paul Starr best described the true measure of how doctors dominated healthcare in America throughout most of its history in America throughout most of its history in his Pulitzer Prize winning book, The Social Transformation of American Medicine.

> "Yet the replacement of a competitive orientation with a corporate consciousness required more than common interests. It required a transfer of power to the group, and this was what began to happen in medicine around 1900 with changes in its social structure. Physicians came increasingly to rely on each other's good will for their access to patients and facilities. Physicians also depended more on their colleagues for defense against malpractice suits, which were increasing in frequency. The courts, in working out the rules of liability for medical practice in the late nineteenth century, had set as the standard of care that of the local community where the physicians practiced. This limited possible expert testimony against physicians to their immediate colleagues. By adopting the "locality rule," the courts prepared the way for granting considerable power to the local medical society, for it became almost impossible for patients to get testimony against a physician who was a member. Medical societies began to make malpractice defense a direct service. Shortly after the turn of the century, doctors in New York, Chicago, and Cleveland organized common defense funds. The Massachusetts Medical Society began handling malpractice suits in 1908. During the next ten years, it supported accused physicians in all but three of the ninety-four cases it received. Only twelve of these ninety-one cases went to trial, all save one resulting in a victory for the doctor. For its first twenty years, the defense fund of the medical society of the state of Washington won every case it fought. Because of their ability to protect their members, medical societies were able to get low insurance rates, while doctors who did not belong could scarcely get any insurance protection. This provided the sort of "selected incentive" that medical societies needed to help them attract members. Professional ostracism carried increasingly serious consequences: denial of hospital privileges, loss of referrals, loss of malpractice insurance, and in extreme cases, loss of a license to practice. The local medical fraternity became the arbiter of a doctor's position and fortune, and he could no longer choose to ignore it. By making the county societies the gate-keeper to membership in any higher professional group, the AMA had recognized and strengthened the position of the local fraternity, as well as bolstering its own organizational underpinnings."

I considered Professor Starr's description of how the AMA controlled the practice of medicine in America 100 years ago similar to the way Al Capone controlled Chicago, the home of the AMA headquarters, for several years, though outright terror.

A department head at the Arnold School of Public Health at the University of South Carolina in Columbia, SC, told me that Professor Starr's book is still required reading at their institution more than thirty years after it was published. Both AMA and Arnold School of Public Health reinforce the understanding that old habits are hard to change.

> "Those who cannot remember the past are
> condemned to repeat it."
>
> ~ George Santayana

But What is Medical Malpractice?

(Depends upon whom you ask.)

Malpractice: Professional misconduct or failure to properly discharge professional duties by failing to meet the standard of care required of a professional.

Unfortunately the American College of Legal Medicine fails to clarify who determines what the "standard of care" is. This shortcoming was rectified in a continuing medical education video presentation made in 2003 by the AMA President-Elect Donald J. Palmisano, MD, JD.

"Doctors, under the law, if you're treating a patient and you fall below a standard of care SET BY THE LAW and those standards are determined by EXPERTS, and that directly causes damage to the patient, that's medical malpractice." [Emphasis mine]

Dr. Palmisano, MD, JD, AMA past-president was the AMA Board representative on the Litigation Center Executive Committee during its creation and in 2002 when Mr. Keene, NCMS general counsel and Bill's Surgeon #2's paths conveniently crossed and allowed the North Carolina Medical Society and Board of Medical Examiners to lead the nation in rooting out nefarious expert witnesses for patients who may have died due to questionable circumstances. But their deaths could not have been due to treatment beneath the clearly recognized standard of care, *set by the law*.

Now for more of Dr. Palmisano's quotes regarding malpractice, litigation, and standard of care.

In his *Need for an Expert* he said, "To determine the standard of care; to determine the height of the "low hurdles" in the race of patient care" . . . "The law requires a MINIMALLY ACCEPTABLE LEVEL OF CARE,

thus my analogy to the "low hurdle".

On PBS, Dr. Palmisano told Ray Suarez, "We do know that the liability system does not measure negligence."

Ray Suarez apparently failed to ask Dr. Palmisano, "Who *does* measure medical negligence?"

Sadly, medical negligence is rarely "measured" by anyone.

AMA brochure, "Will Your Doctor Be There?" (2003), states, "The primary cause of America's medical liability crisis is overzealous personal injury attorneys who put their pocketbooks before patients."

Dr. Palmisano became AMA president in June 2003, and in a two- year period, if we connects the dots, we see that the following events and declarations took place:

- Litigation Center came alive in North Carolina.
- Malpractice is defined as harmful patient care beneath a standard of care *set by the law*.
- Liability system *does not measure* negligence.
- Law *requires a minimally acceptable* level of care.
- Malpractice crisis was (is) *caused by* overzealous attorneys.

What is too easily missed in all of the above? AMA and their constituent state and local societies are like the American Hospital Association and its constituent state members, *associations* (membership organizations), and therefore DEVOID OF AUTHORITY over their respective members.

Note: Dr. Palmisano was the AMA Board member of the Litigation Center Executive Committee with Mr. Keene of the NCMS in 2002.

North Carolina Medical Board, an agency created by the highest power of that state in 1859 and given regulatory authority was necessary to do the AMA-State Medical Societies bidding. No authority is equal to NO REGULATORY ABILITY, and that equals NO ACCOUNTABILITY, even when that accountability appears perhaps to have been misdirected.

By the way: How did attorneys become the "primary cause" of our nation's four-decade-old medical malpractice crisis?

Primary cause is a very important *label* in the practice of medicine. I performed thirty-five autopsies during my six-month Pathology rotation during the second of my three-year oral surgery residency. The *primary purpose* of an autopsy is to identify the *primary cause,* and then also the *secondary causes,* of the death of that deceased patient. Doctors stopped doing autopsies, because they were demonstrating too many inaccurate and poor diagnostic mistakes.

About State Boards of Medical Examiners

Medicine is a regulated profession because of the potential harm to the public if an incompetent or impaired physician is licensed to practice. To protect the public from the unprofessional, improper, unlawful, fraudulent and/or incompetent practice of medicine, each of the fifty states, the District of Columbia, and the US territories has a medical practice act that defines the practice of medicine and *delegates* the *authority* to *enforce the law* to a state medical board.

State medical boards license physicians, investigate complaints, discipline those who violate the law, conduct position evaluations, and facilitate rehabilitation of physicians where appropriate. By following up on complaints, medical boards give the public a way to enforce basic standards of competence and ethical behavior in their physicians, and physicians a way to protect the integrity of their profession. State medical boards also adopt policies and guidelines related to the practice of medicine. There are currently seventy state medical boards authorized to regulate allopathic and osteopathic physicians.

The 10th amendment of the United States Constitution authorizes states to establish laws and regulations protecting the health, safety, and general welfare of their citizens. In response to the tenth amendment, each state legislature enacted a Medical Practice Act that defines the proper practice of medicine and responsibility of the medical board to regulate that practice. [italics emphasis mine]

My Response: Every state's medical board of examiners is more than 100 years old. The paragraphs above may describe the theoretical purpose of such state-created regulatory agencies, but those paragraphs do not describe the reality of how any of those state boards have performed in their attempt to satisfy their original mandate. Try to find even one state board of medical examiners that can provide clear evidence of even coming close to achieving their original mandate.

The AMA-State Medical Societies Litigation Center and the North Carolina Medical Society—North Carolina Medical Board collaboration in 2002 provides a far more accurate picture of medical board efforts to "protect the public." The only state agencies delegated with the authority to regulate the practice of medicine in each and every state have always been missing in action when questionable patient care events occur. That is why hospitals are the only place in America where an accidental death receives NO immediate review by a state source of regulatory authority, and everyone continues to passively accept that sad fact.

A North Carolina physician was appointed to that state's medical board in 2003, the year after that Litigation Center event. That physician became Medical Board president in 2007–2008, and earlier had become involved with the Federation of State Medical Boards in 2005. That earlier committee involvement led to that North Carolina physician being elected to the FSMB Board of Directors in 2008 and ultimately to become the Federation's chairperson for 2011–12.

Federation of State Medical Boards (FSMB)
[from their web site]

> The Federation of State Medical Boards, established in 1912, is a national nonprofit organization representing seventy medical and osteopathic boards within the US and its territories. FSMB started as a small annual gathering of state board executive officers with no permanent staff or headquarters. After more than a century FSMB has grown into a vibrant national organization with nearly 200 employees in Dallas, Texas, and Washington DC.
>
> Vision: The FSMB is a leader in medical regulation, serving as an innovative catalyst for effective policy and standards.

Mission: FSMB promotes excellence in medical practice, licensure, and regulation as a national resource and voice on behalf of state medical boards in their protection of the public.

Values: As an organization of state medical boards, FSMB embraces these equally important values: public protection, leadership, integrity, excellence, and commitment to service.

Will someone ever dare FSMB to provide hard evidence of the above?
FSMB held its 101st anniversary meeting in April 2013 in Boston, Massachusetts.

International Association of Medication Regulatory Authorities (IAMRA)

The Federation of State Medical Boards of the US, under contract with the US Department of Health and Human Services, planned and conducted the first international conference on medical regulation at a meeting in Washington DC in May 1994. Representatives of Australia, Canada, Ireland, New Zealand, South Africa, the United Kingdom, and the United States were in attendance, along with observers from Egypt, Israel, Mexico, and Taiwan.

IAMRA membership list includes over thirty-five national agencies and some of those nations listed include Ghana, India, Indonesia, Kenya, Korea, Malaysia, Nigeria, Pakistan, Sudan, and The Gambia.

The tenth biennial international conference on medical regulation was held in Philadelphia, Pennsylvania in September 2012.

My Response: So the Federation of State Medical Boards and the Department of Health and Human Services felt, almost twenty years ago, and about the time that Harvard School of Public Health researchers were estimating that some 98,000 needless hospital deaths were occurring annually in our hospitals, that all of our state medical boards were doing such a wonderful job in protecting the public, the world could benefit from having an International Association of Medical Regulatory Authorities (note the words *Association* and *regulatory authorities* in that title).

People who complain about the obvious deficiencies in our healthcare delivery system (and most people do complain) need to recognize the need to connect the dots regarding all those who say they are working to make things better in healthcare, and what the evidence clearly demonstrates.

additional insight: This brief, but insightful, article appeared in the *Greenville News* in the early nineties, and about the time the FSMB was helping to create IAMRA.

"Doctors told not to tamper with lawsuit witnesses

South Carolina doctors and their primary insurer will be charged with obstructing justice if they're caught tampering with witnesses in medical malpractice lawsuits from now on. Those who contact witnesses in court cases will risk criminal charges, the US Justice Department warned this week after privately notifying the president-elect of the South Carolina Medical Association that he won't be indicted for talking to a witness last fall.

But that president-elect of the State Medical Association came dangerously close to criminal charges when he urged another doctor to downplay a patient's injuries in court, a letter from federal prosecutors suggests. A similar letter was mailed to the legal counsel for the manager of the Joint Underwriting Association, which insures most doctors in this state. That manager also is the executive director of the patient's compensation fund, which helps pay malpractice verdicts that exceed the Association's $100,000 coverage limit.

The US attorney confirmed that both men are no longer criminal targets but have been put on notice that federal authorities consider any attempt to improperly influence testimony a very serious violation of law, and will be alert to any attempts to cross the lines we have laid down.

The US Justice Department provided that medical society president-elect and that manager of the Joint Underwriting Association, through their attorneys, some stern guidance about the legality of approaching witnesses.

Both men were called before the grand jury after a federal judge heard that they might have tried to influence a doctor's testimony in a three-million-dollar lawsuit. The US attorney refused to disclose the current contents of letters, but he said we made it clear what is legal and what is not in terms of connecting witnesses in any court case.

In the particular instance investigated by the grand jury, based on those facts and circumstances, there was not an illegal attempt to influence a witness under the strict interpretation of the law. We have to consider these things on a case-by-case basis.

Justice Department officials said they expected the medical society president-elect and the manager of the Joint Underwriting Association to spread the word throughout their organizations, however, since both testified in sworn depositions that contacting witnesses has been a common practice for the two associations because of their mutual interest in holding cost of malpractice litigation down.

According to the manager of the Joint Underwriting Association's sworn statement, at least 1000 South Carolina physicians had volunteered to talk to witnesses in such cases, but their purpose is to educate, not intimidate.

~

Everything contained thus far in this chapter was obtained from sources open to the public. At the same time, nothing contained thus far in this chapter would ever see the light of day within any component of the quality of healthcare army of experts.

I have more than fifty years of experience in our nation's healthcare delivery system, and I know that the factual material contained herein thus far raises questions, important questions, that are not only never asked, they are never considered to be asked. Furthermore, the few people who might be capable of asking those important questions would never be allowed to ask them; and even if allowed to ask, they would lack the *authority* sufficient to receive meaningful answers.

Bill's parents merely represent the tip of the tip of the medical malpractice iceberg. The needless hospital death fiasco completely ignores the much larger dilemma of those patients who are, or have received questionable patient care and *lived* to tell the tale. How did our healthcare delivery system come to be such a chaotic mess?

A Brief History of Healthcare

Our healthcare delivery system began the first day a *man* stepped ashore and said, "I am a doctor, and I treat patients." Dr. Benjamin Rush signed the Declaration of Independence in 1776. He was only one of the estimated 3,500 "doctors" in those days. But only one in ten of those "doctors" had obtained a medical degree from a recognized school of medicine.

Doctors initially ruled themselves until organized medicine began to become "organized." And because all doctors are human, and all humans make mistakes, the problem of questionable patient care is, and always will be, an integral part of the "practice" of medicine. Therefore, since doctors (all doctors) will make mistakes, what means are there to respond to those inevitable medical mistakes?

THREE POTENTIAL SYSTEMS

New Jersey Law Revision Commission [from the Medical Peer Review Memorandum] [permission given]

> *Basics of Peer Review*
>
> Medical peer review is a process whereby doctors evaluate the quality of work done by their colleagues, in order to determine compliance with accepted healthcare standards. This self-regulatory procedure provides quality assurance for the medical community by fostering standardization of appropriate medical procedures and by policing caregivers who could pose risks to patients. The rationale for the process is efficiency: working doctors are best situated to judge the competence of other working doctors because they regularly see each others' work and possess the relevant expertise to evaluate it.
>
> A peer review committee typically performs two functions: the initial process of credentialing (reviewing a doctor's qualifications and recommending whether or not the doctor should be granted privileges at the hospital), and ongoing review of a doctor's work within the hospital. Peer review is one of the chief means of monitoring the quality of doctors' work; the other two are state licensing board

disciplinary action and tort law medical malpractice. Ideally, effective peer review should decrease the number of medical malpractice events and improve overall healthcare. Doctors, courts and critics recognize the review process as an efficient means of professional self-regulation. "[P]eer review has become widely accepted as the primary means to weed out low quality physicians and to identify and offer assistance to physicians whose skills need to be enhanced in certain areas." Susan O. Scheutzow, "State Medical Peer Review: High Cost But No Benefit—Is it Time for a Change?" 25 *Am. J. L. & Med.* 7, 15 (1999).

Fundamentals of the review of questionable patient care

The two preceding paragraphs are loaded with what anyone needs to know if they, or a loved one, think they have been harmed by medical care. There are now, and long have been, three, only three, *potential systems* for the review of questionable patient care. Sadly, every one of those potential systems, each for its own reason, has been a miserable failure.

"Ideally, effective peer review should decrease the number of medical malpractice events and improve overall healthcare."

Ideally, our nation should also not be forced to deal with an estimated 200,000 needless hospital deaths annually. Ideal medical peer review, except for a few isolated incidents, has been a figment of organized medicine's imagination, and a tool of their enormous PR. Medical peer review has all of the substance of fog. I know that to be true, and I can prove it.

I served on a hospital formal medical peer review committee in 1976 that took all of the hospital privileges away from a general surgeon who had been in practice in Madison, Wisconsin, for about twenty-five years. This surgeon had been grandfathered into having surgical privileges involving thoracic surgery, vascular surgery, and obstetrical surgery. Unfortunately, that surgeon was having a significantly higher rate of morbidity and mortality complications, because he was continuing to use outdated surgical techniques.

I believe one of the major reasons this surgeon was brought before a medical staff peer review committee was because he had practiced so long in the city in his solo practice, and had never established a support group within his fellow practitioner circle.

Medical peer review, the few times it might take place, rarely involves a doctor well positioned with the in-crowd. Isolated, or fringe members of their local medical community are far more susceptible to being reviewed, should the need arise.

Our peer review committee had no guidelines and no framework to function by, but I believe a majority of that committee's members made the correct decision in removing all of that surgeon's hospital privileges, because he gave every indication that he saw no need in his making any changes in how he treated his patients or why several of his patient care techniques were considered outdated.

That surgeon immediately sued the hospital and each individual member of that review committee for one million dollars each back when one million dollars was big money.

My wife's response was, "What have you got yourself involved in now?" Fortunately, very shortly thereafter a judge denied his suit on the grounds that a hospital medical staff had the right to utilize the peer review process. That ruling meant I could keep my house.

The question that should be asked, and never is, is: does meaningful medical peer review take place within hospital medical staff proceedings on a regular basis throughout our healthcare system? After all, the New Jersey Law Revision Commission said, "Medical peer review is a process whereby doctors evaluate the quality of work done by their colleagues, in order to determine compliance with accepted healthcare standards."

Unfortunately, the answer to, does meaningful medical peer review take place, is, No! Simply put, hospital medical staff peer view occurs about as often as snow falls in New Orleans.

I can offer any state governor and state legislature with a very simple test that could determine the degree of meaningful medical peer review in every hospital in any state—and that process could be rapidly executed. Of course, such a test could only be performed if sufficient authority could be provided. I welcome the challenge to provide such a test, but I am not optimistic that I will ever be able to find a governor or state legislature who might want to know the truth about medical peer review in their state's hospitals. Their citizens would probably like to know, but that is an entirely different matter. Fortunately, this test would not require piercing of the medical peer review veil of secrecy. This last remark however brings up another important point regarding medical peer review.

The Healthcare Quality Improvement Act of 1986 was passed by Congress and contained the intent to protect peer review bodies from private money damage liability—and because organized medicine believed that doctors could not feel free to speak about the patient care of other doctors unless such reports were made in complete secrecy.

I believe organized medicine had an additional reason to seek Congressional passage of an act that would make medical peer review secret, and they were successful in obtaining their ultimate goal. All fifty state legislatures, like lemmings, rapidly followed Congress, and medical peer review is both secret and sacrosanct throughout our nation's hospitals. Unfortunately, due to that impregnable veil of secrecy, meaningful medical peer review's mere existence is left to one's reliance on our medical profession's veracity. Nonetheless, every hospital medical staff leader would respond, if queried, "Certainly we have medical peer review. But I would have to kill you if I told you about it, because medical peer review is secret."

In Chapter 4, I provided the transcript of a conversation between Dr. Wachter and Mr. Boothman. One part of Mr. Boothman's explanation for why their very positive risk management improvements have seemed to hit a plateau fits perfectly here.

"A simple example is a comment that one of our surgeons made to me about two weeks ago. He said to me, 'I was on faculty here six months, at only six months I could give you a short list of people I never wanted to be in an operating room with.' That information is well known. We just need to make greater efforts to tap it and then act on it. Who are those people that everybody knows about who may be unsafe or may be challenged? Maybe we need to get our arms around them and make them safer"

Mr. Boothman goes on to say, "I think that's the next frontier. So what we've managed to do is eliminate the noise. If you think of it as a researcher might, we've eliminated all the variables, but we're down to the cases that are our responsibility. I'm confident we could cut this number yet again by a third, or even a half, just by asking questions that historically we've never asked."

Mr. Boothman then adds, "First of all, interestingly, getting the names is hard. In that conversation I slid a legal pad across the table and I said, "Write them down, and I'll start looking at them," and he wouldn't write them down. There's a complex question about what to do next. First with the culture change: peer review, for instance, has traditionally meant that we wait until somebody bottoms out, until someone has become such an embarrassment or so utterly unsafe that we can't ignore it anymore, then we pluck them out and engage in a very messy and risky process of pulling their privileges or submitting them to a licensing board. That's our shame. We need to get out in front of these people before they become an embarrassment and before they hurt a lot of people. So we're doing a number of things here that are very exciting."

Every hospital medical staff chief in America will tell the public, "Yes, we have medical peer review." Mr. Boothman, however, describes a very accurate picture of the true state of medical peer review in America, and Dr. Makary's quest for *accountability*.

Medical Malpractice Tort Reform

In early March 2004 I was eagerly awaiting, like an expectant father, the arrival of the first copies of my first published book, *First, Do No Harm,* when I noticed in the local paper that a South Carolina Senate Judiciary Subcommittee would be holding a closed hearing regarding tort reform. I attended that closed hearing and joined a gallery of approximately twenty individuals. Their meeting began with about five or six senators seated around the table, and two or three additional senators joined them while the meeting was in progress. Watching those senators seeking to reconcile their widely divergent viewpoints regarding tort reform was like watching middle-aged men herd cats. At the conclusion of that meeting, and after all of the senators left and I was alone in the gallery, I approached the Senate Judiciary Committee's legal counsel and asked him, "How do you maintain your sanity?"

However, there was something beneficial that came out of that chaotic meeting for their future considerations. Tort reform has two distinctly different aspects: commercial and industrial tort reform and medical malpractice tort reform. Just as our healthcare system has two distinctly different aspects (cost and access and healthcare delivery system), all considerations of tort reform, to be effective, must recognize and proceed with that most important understanding. Following that meeting, both Houses of the South Carolina Legislature attempting to deal with tort reform issues had their respective subcommittees separate the two distinctly different aspects of tort reform, and later combine those efforts into a final, legislative bill.

Medical malpractice tort reform has been receiving far more consideration during the last decade than it deserves. Medical malpractice tort reform is the caboose of the medical malpractice litigation system, and that tort reform aspect can only become viable IF the plaintiff (patient) wins their case against the doctor, which only occurs statistically in about one out of ten medical malpractice trials. Medical malpractice tort reform is no magic wand, and it never has been.

To understand medical malpractice tort reform, one must first understand medical malpractice litigation. To understand medical malpractice litigation, one must first understand medical malpractice. I repeat, I detest the term "medical malpractice" because it is a pejorative and assumes a negative before any negative has been confirmed.

Questionable patient care review, fair to both doctor and patient, should be the goal sought regardless of which of the three potential systems of questionable patient care review are being used. Unfortunately, organized medicine, over a century and a half ago, led our nation and its leaders to passively accept medical malpractice litigation (Sue or forget it), as the system of choice for the review of questionable patient care. Our medical profession and the public have been paying a huge price for that unprofessional decision ever since.

Mr. Boothman, in his conversation with Dr. Wachter, clearly expressed his disdain for that system that he recognized early in his career as a medical malpractice trial lawyer. When trial lawyers recognize that civil litigation should not be the system of choice for the review of questionable patient care, people should take notice. But there is more about how the consistent drumbeat for more and better medical malpractice tort reform is purposely ignoring the facts.

The Congressional Budget Office (CBO) estimated that up to fifty billion dollars could be saved in our healthcare system in a decade with more medical malpractice tort reform. I'd had a very cordial conversation with a person at the CBO in 2008 regarding medical malpractice and an article he had contributed to regarding that subject. Therefore when I saw the latest CBO estimate of a potentially enormous savings due to medical malpractice tort reform, I called that individual again. I asked him who came up with this figure, and he said he did. I said there was absolutely no way this could be possible, or even justified with hard accounting data over time. We continued with another very cordial conversation about tort reform and other healthcare issues, but he could provide no specifics on how one might be able to arrive at a more accurate estimate.

CBO staff, I believe, function like galley slaves. Members of Congress send them specific requests for financial estimates; and those CBO staff members are required to provide those estimates even if, or when, those congressional requests make no sense. CBO estimates are like playing poker with a person who is dealing with their own marked cards. There cannot be, and will not be, billions of dollars saved due to federal medical malpractice tort reform.

Experts have failed to recognize that there is a perfect example however of how one might hope to calculate possible medical malpractice tort reform savings and how those previous calculations of potential savings have never materialized. Let me explain.

During George W. Bush's first term, organized medicine determined that the time was ripe due to the presence of a Republican president and a Republican-controlled Congress to push for strong medical malpractice tort reform in Congress. AMA, in 2003, published a sixty-page proposal entitled "Tort Reform—Now!" Well into the body of that manuscript, they provided a perfect method for someone to truly judge the financial and patient safety benefits of medical malpractice tort reform.

California Medical Injury Compensation Reform Act–75 (MICRA-75) was reported in the AMA proposal "Tort Reform—Now" as being the gold standard for medical malpractice tort reform. This AMA declaration provides the perfect way to truly judge the long-term benefits of medical malpractice tort reform for two reasons:

First, ask if the citizens of California have enjoyed significantly more patient safety due to MICRA-75 than those citizens of all of the other states who have been denied such a medical malpractice tort reform gold standard since 1975. The answer is NO!

Second, considering the thirty-eight-year time span between the passage of MICRA-75 and the AMA Tort Reform-Now declaration in 2003, someone in California should be able to provide the mathematical formula used to determine the amount saved in that state due to the AMA gold standard for medical malpractice tort reform.

There is no formula, and there never has been. Doctor's malpractice insurance premiums may go down slightly, or stay unchanged for a while, but calculable savings, or increased patient safety never becomes evident. The South Carolina Legislature has been dealing with tort reform issues in every two-year legislative cycle since 2004. See if they can say how much money has been saved due to all of their tort reform efforts all these years. The public needs to understand that every time anyone, regardless of their degree of healthcare expertise, cries for greater medical malpractice tort reform, they are at the same time telling the public: you will continue to be left with "Sue or forget it," because medical malpractice tort reform is merely the caboose of the medical malpractice litigation system. Also, medical malpractice tort reform *only becomes activated* in the few (one out of ten) cases where the plaintiff (patient) wins the case. We have seen through the unfortunate circumstances of the highly questionable death of Bill and the workings of the AMA—50 States Medical Society—State Medical Board collaboration that organized medicine's priorities place the welfare of the doctors before the welfare of patients who may have been harmed by questionable patient care.

Organized Medicine's Two Faces

Review the *Journal of the American Medical Association (JAMA)* published from 1949–2003, as I did; and you will see the two faces of organized medicine, each one in stark contrast to the other. Initially, the AMA leadership said all of the right things as best illustrated by this quote:

In *JAMA* in October 1958: "What marks a profession? It is obligated to assure the public of the competence of its members and the quality of their work. It is obligated to assume the responsibility of disciplining those who do not measure up to the accepted ethical practices of the profession? Only physicians can judge the competence of their colleagues and can prohibit the kinds of conduct harmful to patients and the profession."

That dramatic soliloquy is precisely what the word "profession" implies, and what every patient has always assumed they could hope to receive. That quote, while speaking volumes, is only one of many such quotes issued by the AMA in the early years of the new "era of modern medicine" following WWII. Unfortunately, for both sides of the medical equation, the AMA's eloquent rhetoric became hollow promises.

Compare and Contrast

Earlier in this chapter, I talked about how a Surgery Specialty Department chairman at the local University of Wisconsin Medical School and Hospital had lied in his sworn testimony in his deposition regarding the first surgeon's ability to meet an acceptable standard of care. In my expert witness testimony to the Special Medical Malpractice Panel hearing that case, I testified as the second surgeon that that patient had been "surgically mutilated."

At the end of 1984 I was removed from being a member of the Oral Surgery Group that I joined in 1966, because of my activities as an expert witness in cases where I was the second surgeon. I had not sought out that responsibility, but I did feel it was my ethical and professional responsibility to answer questions asked by those with a right to ask them. I was well aware that I was breaking the "Code of Silence," but I could not refuse to provide the detailed information that only a second surgeon is best able to provide in cases involving gross malpractice, as two of my cases did.

Therefore, in early 1985, I opened a solo practice on the West side of Madison, Wisconsin. Federally initiated HMOs had become a major presence by that time in Madison, Wisconsin; yet I was the only board certified oral and maxillofacial surgeon who was denied an opportunity to be accepted as a practitioner in four of the five local HMOs. My ability to grow a viable solo practice was greatly limited.

The surgeon who surgically mutilated that patient continued unabated to practice his rather outdated forms of surgery. Within five years, I, the second surgeon who broke the "Code of Silence," would be economically put out of business and forced to leave the state. But prior to that, I made a major decision that would redirect my life and ultimately lead me to writing this, my third book on our healthcare delivery system.

In January 1986, after a great deal of soul-searching, I made the decision to become an expert regarding medical malpractice and "Sue or forget it." In order to do that, I felt that I had to begin to advertise nationally that I was available to provide expert witness testimony. That was not an easy decision to make, but one I have never regretted. There are a lot of "dirty jobs" throughout the way we do business in this country, and becoming a medical malpractice expert witness is one of them.

My very first case has great similarity with what happened in that previous case in Madison, Wisconsin, involving that surgically mutilated patient. I received a phone call from an attorney in Columbus, Ohio, who was representing a middle-aged woman who had in all appearances received substandard care from an oral surgeon in that city who was also a part-time faculty member of the Oral Surgery Department at the Ohio State University, and an officer in the Regional Great Lakes Oral Surgery Society.

After receiving the files, photographs, and x-rays involved in that patient's case, and reviewing them, I called that attorney and said this patient's treatment was so substandard that I assumed that oral surgeon would not even consider going to trial. It was obvious to me, and should have been obvious to everyone else with any understanding regarding the surgical correction of jaw deformities, that the surgeon was completely unqualified for even attempting such a surgical procedure. I could not have been more wrong in my assumption!

Chairman of the Oral and Maxillofacial Surgery Department at the Wisconsin Medical School in Milwaukee testified under oath in his deposition that he believed the first surgeon had provided a reasonable standard of care. That patient's attorney contacted me and said that he did not believe they could overcome that testimony from such a high level professional source, and therefore they were dropping their activity in pursuing this case further.

People must be aware that pursuing litigation in medical malpractice cases creates a major financial burden on both the attorneys and the patients involved, particularly when it is recognized that patients win their cases in, at best, one out of ten malpractice trials. To my knowledge, that surgically harmed patient never received her day in court for two reasons: that Surgery Department chairman's misleading testimony, and the additional fact that her second surgeon, an MD/DDS in Columbus, Ohio, told her he would surgically correct her existing facial deformity, but he would not testify against the first surgeon. The Code of Silence won again.

I confronted that Oral Surgery Department chairman and defense expert witness at an oral surgery conference a few months after I had had an opportunity to read his deposition. I asked him how he could testify under oath in such a clearly untrue manner. He replied that he did not have all of the records when he gave his deposition, which had to be an additional lie to go along with his misleading deposition testimony. Then he hastily walked away and avoided me for the rest of the conference.

Thankfully, I still don't know how so many "professionals" can disregard their ethical obligation so easily; but such behavior is, and has been, a major characteristic of our healthcare professions—easily recognized, but continually ignored by most, but not all.

"The Professions Under Siege", Jacques Barzun, Harper's Magazine, October 1978.

I was led to this article by an editorial in the *Journal of the American Dental Association* in October 1984. That editorial led me to go to the local library and copy that article and always have one or more copies close at hand. Here are a few quotes from that insightful article.

A profession is an institution, and as such it cuts a figure in public that may or may not match the prevailing habits and merits of the practitioners. The insiders genuinely believe in that figure; they live by it in more ways than one, and they can hardly help thinking of the profession as going on forever in the same glorious way, altering itself only as it improves performance by new skill.

According to Dr. Abraham Flexner, the famous critic and reformer of medical education fifty years ago, to be medically trained implies the possession of certain portions of many sciences arranged and organized with a distinct practical purpose in view. That is what makes it a profession. The key words here are: a distinct practical purpose in view, for which special training is required. Since the laity, by definition, has no such purposes and lack special training, a profession is necessarily a monopoly. In modern societies, this monopoly is made legal by a license to practice; but the professions have always managed to form a guild, a trade union, claiming the exclusive right to practice the art. But between monopoly and conspiracy the line of demarcation is hard to fix and easy to step over.

What every professional should bear in mind is the distinction between a profession and a function. The function may well be the eternal; but the profession, which is the cluster of practices and relationships arising from the function at a given time and place, can be destroyed—or can destroy itself—very rapidly.

The modern professions have enjoyed their monopoly for so long that they have forgotten that it is a privilege given in exchange for a public benefit.

But what the professions need in their present predicament is, first, the will to police themselves with no fraternal hand, with no thought of public relations. Any few scandals giving the group a bad name will soon convince the public that self-policing means what it says and confidence will return. Screening and disciplining from within must always continue, steadily and firm, or it will be taken over by public bodies and officialdom.

English has borrowed from French the phrase *esprit de corps* and uses it to mean something good—team spirit, loyalty. But in French, to this day, it means something bad: the huddling together of members of the guild to hush up their mistakes; it means in short, Shaw's conspiracy against the laity. (Bernard Shaw said, "Every profession is a conspiracy against the laity.")

Policing, being negative, is not enough. It will not effect moral regeneration, which can come about only when the members of a group feel once more confident that ethical behavior is desirable, widely practiced, approved, and admired.

What all professions need today is critics from inside, men who know what the conditions are, and also the arguments and excuses, and in a full sweep over the field can offer their fellow practitioners a new vision of the profession as an institution.

He nailed it! The first time I read "The Professions Under Siege" almost thirty years ago, I thought: here is a man with no medical training, but one who sees clearly what is, and has been, taking place within our healing professions; and they can't hear him, or more likely, refuse to listen. Since first reading that article, I have hoped I might someday become one of those "critics from inside, men who know what the conditions are, and also the arguments and excuses, and in a full sweep over the field can offer their fellow practitioners a new vision of the profession as an institution." Jacques Barzun finished writing *From Dawn to Decadence: 500 Years of Western Cultural Life* (877 pages) in 2000 and at age ninety-two. Professor Barzun passed away in November 2012 at the age of 104.

That earlier *JAMA* October 1958 article, "What marks a profession?," quote mirrors Professor Barzun's description—so we know that "they knew" what a true profession demands of its members. But unfortunately, they have always been able to "talk the talk," while lacking the ability to "walk the walk."

Now I feel I must "walk the walk" and raise a question that must be asked. I just wish someone else would ask the question, but I know without a doubt that if I don't ask it, no one else ever will. I am qualified to ask the question, but I do not have the ability to answer this question that I feel should be asked and answered.

Has AAOMS Crossed the Line?

I was so proud to become a member of the American Association of Oral and Maxillofacial Surgeons (AAOMS), and Wisconsin delegate to several annual House of Delegates, presenter at Scientific Sessions, and Wisconsin State president of our state society. But I was not too proud to raise questions and initiate beneficial change regarding the relationship between the AAOMS, as parent organization, and the American Board of Oral and Maxillofacial Surgeons after I became Board Certified. As Professor Barzun pointed out, professions need critics from within, and I have been such on several occasions. But this next issue goes far beyond any issue I could ever imagine.

Some clarifications are necessary:

American Association of Oral and Maxillofacial Surgeons (AAOMS) is the parent organization.

OMS National Insurance Company (OMSNIC) is an AAOMS-created malpractice insurance source that collaborates with a malpractice insurance company.

OMS indicates individual oral and maxillofacial surgeons who are insured by OMSNIC.

Fortress Insurance Company underwrites the malpractice insurance as a subsidiary of OMSNIC.

Note: Copyright permission for use of unaltered excerpts from the OMSNIC Monitor, (a quarterly newsletter), copies of which I have been receiving as a retired Fellow (board certified member) of AAOMS through the years, was verbally denied by an OMSNIC in-house attorney, and understandably so. The unaltered excerpts I had taken and hoped to use from only three Monitor issues during the period between 2010 -2012 were sufficient for me to question the propriety of how a major surgical specialty has actively immersed itself into the malpractice protection business of its members. Thus, the following, sanitized description of AAOMS/OMSNIC activities on behalf of their members will lack the clarity this subject deserves.

AAOMS created OMSNIC in 1988 and that in-house malpractice insurance middleman will celebrate its 25th anniversary in 2013 under a quid pro quo arrangement with financial benefits to both entities. OMSNIC promotes itself as a professional liability insurance company that aggressively defends its members subject to claims of negligent patient care. One Monitor issue went into great detail regarding the standard of care, a breach of same, and the duties and obligations of an expert witness during malpractice litigation proceedings.

One quote in the August 2011 issue is what has led me to strongly consider including this segment in Find The Black Box: oral surgeons who wish to serve as expert witnesses *must not do so in cases for which they also served as one of the patient's treating doctors.*

Monitor August 2012 issue left me with what I feel to be no choice: In that issue OMSNIC describes their 10th Defense Counsel Seminar, in conjunction with Fortress Insurance Company in honoring well-over one hundred attorneys from across America who have valiantly serve that surgical specialty in defending insured members faced with malpractice litigation. And that issue provided a graft diagram to illustrate just how successful those defense attorneys had been performing in courts.

Well, you tell me: has my surgical specialty, AAOMS, crossed the line legally? I believe, without question, they have gone far beyond the ethical and true profession lines.

In all of the cases I have ever been involved with, but particularly in those cases where I testified as the second surgeon, NO ONE at either hospital EVER ASKED: how is the patient? In the first case that occurred at the Catholic hospital in Madison, WI., I made sure that I ascended in the proper order, from bottom to top, every medical staff and administration committee, including the Medical Staff Committee, Executive Committee, chief administrator, and even the Sister House in St. Louis. NO ONE cared to ask about the patient!

One more piece of the medical malpractice puzzle

What happens when a needless hospital death involves a loved one of a member of the medical profession? This next article will take the reader into just such a scenario.

Note: The substance of this next brief story of one more of the 200,000 needless hospital deaths occurring annually was obtained second hand from its original source, our nation's premier healthcare policy journal. I declined to pay a four-figure royalty to quote the article in its entirety (seven pages without references) IF it only appeared in an eBook format, and an undisclosed additional sum if it appeared in a print format. I do not say this to denigrate that journal's editorial decision makers. They run a business and they and their staff must be paid. That said, I have tried to include a few articles in their entirety so that those readers with sufficient interest can have access to a few samples in order to see "What they say and how they say it" and also in "What they don't say and how they seem to consistently miss some of the most important points each story provides.

Mother's dying, Someone do Something!

An abundance of tragic stories involving medical errors can be found in all forms of the media including healthcare journals and that should not be surprising considering the fact that there is estimated to be 200,000 needless hospital deaths annually. Most of those stories, unfortunately, have several similarities in that they speak of the many ways that medical errors may occur and also of the dysfunctional approach typically taken in response to those errors. The very important aspect of how to respond to medical errors in a concise and organized manner is rarely, if ever mentioned. I include one such tragic story of a medical error because this never event involves both a treating doctor and a practicing physician and close relative of the unfortunate patient on each side of the medical dilemma.

There are three major players in this tragic story, Mother, Doctor/ Oncologist and Doctor/Son. The event took place in a Midwestern state where Doctor/ Son's parents continued to reside and where he had grown up. At the time of the event however Doctor/ Son was practicing medicine at a medical center located in a major city on the East Coast.

Mother had been diagnosed with cancer and treated by Doctor/ Oncologist initially over ten years earlier and had gone into remission. Unfortunately, Mother was diagnosed with a recurrence of her cancer and evidence of its spread to another part of her body in close proximity to the site of her original lesion two years before the event in question here took place. Doctor/Oncologist had resumed medical responsibility for this episode of patient care and her current treatment seemed to be affective – until the event of this story.

Doctor/Son received a call from an ER doctor at his hometown hospital because his father had rushed Mother to that hospital in critical condition. As that ER doctor described Mother's condition Doctor/Son knew exactly what her immediate problem was and precisely what treatment protocol she needed. Doctor/Son is a practicing ER physician, and in that capacity he is often the first doctor to see and evaluate patients entering his ER with similar, urgent need for immediate care, therefore he knew what Mother needed and that she MUST receive all of the elements of that treatment protocol within the next 24 hours for it to be successful. Doctor/Son told that ER doctor to tell his family that he would leave immediately and be there as soon as possible.

Doctor/Son arrived twelve hours later and found, much to his dismay, that the treatment protocol his Mother desperately needed had not been ordered, therefore not started, and Doctor/Oncologist had gone home. Doctor/Son sent his family members home and he remained at Mother's bedside, watching, waiting and hoping that something or someone would do something positive, but this would not have become another never event if such had taken place.

Doctor/Son finally, at midnight, demanded that Mother be moved to ICU, thinking that an ICU physician would immediately recognize Mother's critical condition, her urgent need, and begin the desperately needed and well established treatment protocol that was necessary to get her through her current crisis. Mother was moved to ICU, and NOTHING HAPPENED!

Doctor/Son was informed by an ICU nurse that their doctors could not begin new patient care treatments until and unless the patient's primary care physician had given permission, but Doctor/Oncologist was home in bed. To make matters worse, if possible, Doctor/Son was told by the ICU nurse that they did have the treatment protocol Mother so desperately needed, BUT Doctor/Oncologist had not ordered it. In the 23rd hour of Mother's critical 24 hour window that treatment protocol was started. Several days later Mother died. Where does that tragic event leave Doctor/ Son and his family?

Sue or forget it! Yes, even Doctor/Son, Doctor/Son's Doctor/Wife and their medical colleagues back at the medical center on the East Coast were "forced" to consider the unthinkable. Ultimately Doctor/Son and his family could not bring themselves to cross that line, even though Doctor/ Son's profession had been leaving Society with that dilemma throughout the entire history of their profession.

The article continues to spend as much consideration regarding that hospital's administration and medical staff's tepid response to that never event as it does to the event itself, but there is one additional decision worth of comment. Doctor/Son's resolve to forget it rather than sue was made with a consensus between he and the hospital medical staff leaders that Doctor/Oncologist was nearing retirement and such a suit would stain his long career. There was no mention in the article about how that hospital medical staff might react if Doctor/Oncologist was to repeat that patient- care failure and initiate one, or even more, additional similar never events. Doctors and hospital medical staffs seem to always make these decisions about lapses in sound medical judgment without ever thinking about their responsibility to the community they seek to serve.

This article, and very sad story, contains a graphic picture of our current healthcare delivery system—AND—its fundamental dysfunction due to the absence of an organizational structure with clearly defined points of *authority, delegated authority,* and any opportunity for *meaningful accountability.*

Most of the estimated 200,000 needless hospital deaths do not include a doctor as part of the collateral damage. We have heard about the very positive improvements at the University of Pittsburgh Medical Center, Mr. Boothman's risk management improvements at the University of Michigan Health System (where he can't identify certain "questionable surgeons"), University of Washington Medical Center, and the Agency for Healthcare Research and Quality (AHRQ).

But no one talks about:
- States who license doctors—and who regulates hospitals?
- State medical examining boards, mandated to "regulate the practice of medicine.
- Surgery centers, where needless deaths also, occasionally, take place.
- Accountability, and its presence, anywhere in each state's healthcare delivery system.
- "Sue or forget it" being the system of choice for the review of questionable patient care.

That list could go on. Even doctors are forced to consider malpractice litigation, but only if where they practice is far removed from the site of questionable patient care. This family had their own fully qualified expert witness. But doctors know they must never cross that line; they must remain acceptable to all other members of their "profession."

As a doctor in a high-risk field, Doctor/Son considered how destructive a malpractice suit could be if they sued Doctor/Oncologist. He would be a central figure in the case, as the debacle fell squarely in his lap. He was imperfect, but his mother had respected him. He was nearing retirement, and a lawsuit would be a terrible way to end his career. Doctor/Son didn't want to do that to him, even though he'd never explained his inaction. As a physician Doctor/Son felt an odd empathy; a lawsuit would desecrate his years of service. They had to find an alternative. A lawsuit just wasn't in line with their Midwestern family mindset.

But, what if this older doctor repeats this tragedy on another patient? What would that hospital administration and medical staff tell that patient's family? There is a much better way for hospital medical staff's to handle these type situations, but that way will require doctors to fairly judge other doctors, and not many doctors can even consider ever doing that.

I believe this sad story illustrates, in great detail, what is missing, and what has always been missing in our nation's healthcare delivery system. Yet no one within the quality of healthcare army of experts has ever given the slightest bit of recognition or consideration regarding the state's (every state's) responsibility for their obligation to all of their citizens in our nation's entire healthcare delivery system.

~

Each reader, hopefully there will be some, must decide for themselves what Chapters 3-5 says to them about their, and their children's and grandchildren's healthcare delivery system, and also about how the various components of our nation's medical and dental professions are conducting themselves, and how productive the efforts of that enormous army of quality of healthcare experts have been in creating meaningful change and greater patient safety.

MADD, in my opinion, is the role model for those who accept as dual facts, all medical care is local and state's license doctors; therefore states are responsible for their state's healthcare delivery system. Like MADD, if you want state governors and legislators to respond to your demands for meaningful change, you must unite in sufficient numbers to threaten their possibility for re-election (their individual priority #1).

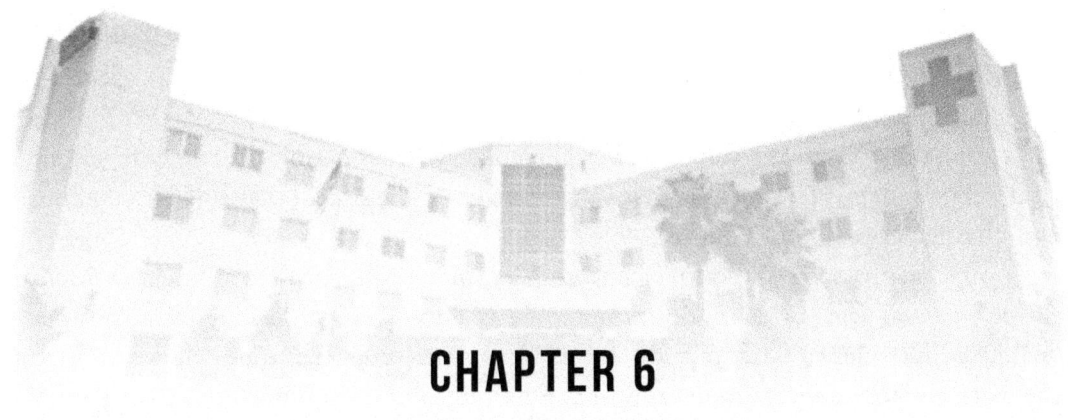

CHAPTER 6

WHAT A COLLAGE OF BOOK REVIEWS TELLS US

According to the *2013 Guide to Literary Agents*, books with the subject of healthcare primarily fall under one of two categories: Health and Medicine. Few people, I presume, are able to read every book that comes out in both of those categories, but I have always felt it important to read those that were authored by healthcare experts that appear to be seeking the same goal I seek: an opportunity to make our healthcare delivery system far better.

Authors are faced with the question of "who is your audience?" and "what makes your book different?" Because my perspective on the root cause of the plethora of problems within our healthcare system is so different from that of any other source I am familiar with, I face no difficulty in presenting how my book differs from practically any other book on healthcare thus far. At the same time, my iconoclastic views have made my efforts to secure an audience, for all practical purposes, difficult. Machiavelli and Semmelweis provide clues to my problems in that regard.

I have always believed that anyone writing a non-fiction book on a serious subject should seek to respond to what should be anticipated criticism. I've made great efforts in the past to make my books available to those I considered, and who are recognized as, experts in the quality of healthcare field. I can only speculate as to why the dozens of such experts, after assuring me of their willingness to accept a copy, have provided me with no response whatsoever. I have always hoped these individuals would share their comments, both positive and negative. The single brief exception was Dr. Wachter's reply email regarding *Misdiagnosed*: "You make some important points and I agree that peer review is a critical, and mostly neglected, component of patient safety."

This "books" chapter is included to reinforce the need to read multiple books, articles, and news releases in order to begin to connect the dots and gain a deeper insight into how totally unorganized and dysfunctional "your" healthcare delivery system truly is. Not one single, or even a couple, of these books, including mine, can convey the depth of the fundamental problems throughout our nation's healthcare delivery system.

I hope this collective review and well-intended critiques permit the reader to see more clearly the fundamental flaws that have always afflicted the system that will directly impact every living person in our nation.

I offer, in the spirit of courtesy and respect, my critique of several books written in the past several years by those I presume to be as sincere as I am in their efforts to make healthcare in America far better. Books on serious subjects need to be "chewed on," and there are few topics more important, or more in need of deep discussion, than the trials and tribulations of our current healthcare system.

Hopefully, excerpts from this collection of books, coupled with the offering contained in "Sue or forget it" will provide a composite picture of "our" healthcare delivery system.

Can't Is Not an Option by Nikki Haley, Governor of South Carolina

Note: I had hoped to include 8 brief quotes (172 total words) taken without alteration from my state governor's nationally acclaimed book, but permission was denied by a failure to respond to my multiple requests. There was nothing new or radically different about her quotes because they merely indicated her personal desire to solve problems, make people's lives better, seek challenges, provide accountability, work for the people of South Carolina, and to seek people dedicated to reforming our state. I will leave my response to those eight simple quotes I had hoped to include unchanged.

My Response

Governor Haley, I believe, is a very honest and sincere person/politician, and in her book she says all the right things. In my review of *JAMA* articles while preparing to write my first book, I found that each new AMA president's annual letter to the members printed in the *JAMA* also said all the right things: "Doctors, we must judge other doctors," "If we don't do it someone else will," "We owe it to the public," and on and on. But well-spoken intentions become mere platitudes when that intent fails to become action. AMA gave the public their Litigation Center instead.

Dr. Spence Taylor, chairman of the Department of General Surgery at Greenville Memorial Hospital and operations director of the USC School of Medicine/Greenville Developmental Team, in his very pristine assessment in April 2010, accurately described the state of South Carolina's healthcare delivery system when he said, "Even if you cured cancer, you couldn't get it to the people, because the medical system is broken." Yet his accurate description of the current state of affairs regarding the state's healthcare delivery system appeared to go in one ear and out the other of every decision maker in the state.

I see two major obstacles for any state's decision makers to adequately confront their sad state of affairs within their state healthcare delivery system:

1. The "cost and access" aspect of healthcare dominates the thinking of practically every decision maker at the federal and state level throughout our nation. What such single-minded thinking obscures is the fact that they seek to save *money* by changing that cost and access aspect of healthcare while not realizing that they can save both *lives and money* by creating an organizational structure for their healthcare delivery system.
2. The failure at both the federal and state level to recognize the full meaning of the word *authority*, and the use of *delegated authority* in order to create meaningful *accountability*. There is no doubt in my mind that, if I could find one governor and legislature to join together and provide me with sufficient delegated authority to act as their tool and provide me with an opportunity to give them a complete, detailed picture of their current healthcare delivery system, their state would become the role model for every other state.

Most, perhaps all, state governors say, and believe, similar ideas as those conveyed by Governor Haley. But, unless each governor and state legislature can ever come to recognize the two equally important, but distinctly different, aspects of healthcare (cost and access AND healthcare delivery system), chaos will continue to reign in their state's healthcare system and continue to deny their citizens what they deserve.

Unaccountable: What Hospitals Won't Tell You and How Transparency Can Revolutionize Healthcare, Marty Makary, MD.

Note: Stark contrast: Dr. Makary did rapidly respond to my request for permission to use excerpts from his book. The title of his book, Unaccountable, sums up the state of our nation's healthcare delivery system in one word, and that word illustrates why 200,000 needless hospital deaths continue unabated, in spite of enormous effort by so many experts who have never recognized the importance of the full meaning of that word.

Selected excerpts:

> A hospital is no longer the community pillar I knew growing up, with its altruistic mission guiding its decisions. Hospitals have merged and transformed into giant corporations with little accountability—and they like it that way.
>
> In 2010 a Harvard study published in the prestigious *New England Journal of Medicine* reported a finding well-known to medical professionals: as many as 25 percent of all patients are harmed by medical mistakes. What's even less known to the public is that over the past ten years, error rates have not come down, despite numerous efforts to make medical care safer.
>
> Dr. Lucian Leape, at a national surgeon's conference opened the gathering's keynote speech by looking out over the audience of thousands and asking the doctors to "raise your hand if you know of a physician you work with who

should not be practicing because he or she is dangerous." Every hand went up. Incredulous at this response, I took to asking the same question whenever I spoke at conferences. And I always got the same response. Every doctor knows about this problem— but few talk about it. Every day, people are injured or killed by medical mistakes that might have been prevented with a modicum of adherence to standardize guidelines. The silence about the problem has paralyzed efforts to address it—until now. Medicine is its own culture. It has its own language, ethos, and code of justice. Doctors swear to do no harm. But on the job they soon absorb another unspoken rule: to overlook malpractice in their colleagues.

We all know the healthcare system is broken, burdening our families, businesses, and national debt. It needs common-sense reform.

The patients whose numbers came up with Dr. Hodad were just the unlucky victims of a system lacking in standardization, oversight, or ways to measure quality.

But watching Hodad in action made me realize that patient satisfaction was only half the story. Patients couldn't know what we staff in the operating room could see: that the man was dangerous, had poor judgment, and practice outdated medicine. Doctors work in a disjointed system with perverse incentives, little oversight, and a lot of haggling that goes on behind closed doors far from public view—kind of like Congress.

There were other, more powerful ways I was "educated" on the code of silence. Once in a hospital peer review conference, I witnessed the futility of a brave doctors speaking up to condemn another doctor's careless decision to operate when the operation didn't meet criteria. The doctor at fault gave a justification that a courtroom would believe, but we all knew it was not true. It was a rare spectacle, yet nothing came out of it, except that the brave doctor who spoke up became a marked man. Throughout my training, I witnessed several doctors run out of town because their honesty and outspokenness begin to poke the bear. In many ways, direct and indirect, I was taught that the code of silence was part of being a doctor.

Unlike aviation, hundreds of thousands of lives are lost each year due to preventable mistakes by doctors.

If we had more of it, the accountability visited on hospitals would revolutionize the quality of medical care in every city in America, dramatically reshaping our healthcare landscape.

Seeking accurate ways to measure patient outcomes has long been the holy grail of healthcare reform, the starting point for fixing our broken healthcare system.

As I listen to Dr. Leape talk about secret addictions and other common impairments, I realized that he wasn't just talking about doctors who simply have poor skills or bad judgment. This was an entirely different problem. He was talking about doctors affected by dependence problems and other physical and mental impairments. That's when the problem of impaired physicians struck me as nothing less than a public health crisis. I did some more math. If, say, only 2 percent of the nation's one million doctors are seriously impaired by drugs, alcohol abuse, or other major impairments (and most experts agree that 2 percent is a low estimate), that means twenty thousand impaired doctors are practicing medicine. I asked, "What can be done about these few bad apples affecting so many people?" Dr. Leape smiled, and said, "The state medical boards take care of that."

Yet there are also grossly impaired physicians, doctors with horrible skills, hazardous judgment, ulterior motives, or who suffer from substance abuse or other problems that make them dangerous. Society ought to be able to deal with this better, not sweep it all under the rug. Doctoring is a stressful profession with easy access to drugs, so it's no mystery why doctors have substance abuse problems. In fact, rates of serious substance abuse and psychiatric disease among doctors are actually higher than that of other professions with similar educational background and socioeconomic status.

In my original calculation estimating the magnitude of the impaired physician problem, I estimated that 2 percent of doctors are impaired. However .... I agree with others that 2 percent is a drastic understatement of the true incidence of impaired physicians.

One time, right after this notoriously bad surgeon's run of six deaths, my friend was administrating anesthesia for him. In front of all the operating room nurses and technicians, the patient asked my friend before going off to sleep, "Is my surgeon a good surgeon?" The operating room staff froze as their eyes popped out of their heads. They stared at my friend to see how he would deal with the direct question. "He's one of the four best heart surgeons we have here," he said with a smile. Luckily for my friend, the patient didn't follow up with, "And how many heart surgeons do you have here?"

Having inside knowledge about a risky doctor while trying to comfort his patient in preparation for surgery is a dilemma every healthcare provider knows all too well. I asked my friend if he ever thought about reporting this surgeon to someone. He laughed and asked, "Like who?"

The hospital administration loved this young heart surgeon, who was making a financial killing (pardon the pun) off his work. The senior partners were very protective of him as the youngest member of their group—after all, he took most of their weekend calls for them. He covered their holiday shifts and happily tended to whatever the senior surgeons did not like to do, such as operating on their obese patients for them. They cut the young doc tremendous slack whenever his complications were discussed at a peer review conference, saying a patient's death was attributable to some extenuating patient circumstances. (That's right, they'd blame the victim.) Such internal peer reviews are a little like the Russian parliament under Stalin. No matter how much discussion there is, the result seems foreordained. At these internal peer review conferences, complicated cases are reduced to biased two-to- three-minute summaries, and doctors who might raise probing questions are well aware that they can pay a heavy price for challenging their peers.

Doctors and nurses know of docs who are reckless, but it takes moving a mountain to do something about it. Not reporting incompetence among peers is part of medical culture and has been for centuries. Medicine is poorly policed.

How about the national doctors associations? Can they police their own time? As a member of several, only once have I ever heard of a program that tried to address impaired physicians, and that effort never picked up steam. After asking around, it became clear that the only time that a doctors association would ever consider taking action against the doctor was if a state medical board had already done so. Hungry to grow their membership and collect annual dues, doctors associations are historically passive when it comes to policing doctors (the AMA is actively recruiting to increase its membership, which is now declined to 15 percent of US doctors; membership cost $420 a year). Policing doctors is a job so messy no one wants to do it. So who is in charge of policing medical care in America?

Every organization, institution, medical association, and hospital administrator that I have asked has told me that policing physicians is the real responsibility of state medical boards. So let's examine the role of state medical boards in American medicine.

State medical boards

Consider California. The Medical Board of California, like all others, is responsible for licensing and disciplining physicians. On three different audits conducted during the 1980s, the California attorney general found that the board wasn't doing its job. Apart from that announcement, no further action was taken. The board went eighteen years without another audit until 2003, when University of San Diego Law School Professor Julie D'Angelo Fellmeth became the medical board enforcement monitor. Then she blew a whistle. Testifying to a Senate committee in 2008 after years of trying to sound alarms, she said the Medical Board of California "routinely failed to promptly remove from work physician participants who tested positive for prohibited substances." The board had five out of five failed audit audits. Julie D'Angelo Fellmeth was let go. The Medical Board of California then went on doing whatever it does about impaired physicians, which is to say, not much.

Impaired physicians are a small minority of doctors who are very destructive and difficult to police. Knowingly or unknowingly, they cause a lot of harm. State medical boards are sometimes aware of them, but look the other way. Standards for doctors are local and vary widely state by state.

Nearly every doctor can name a doctor who needs to retire but won't—impaired doctors in their nineties who refused to leave the office even when they are no longer being paid. Why do we have this problem? The reason is there are no rules.

I can legally do anything. In fact, some varicose vein removal centers in the United States are run by former OB/ GYN doctors, and others by psychiatrists; they were doctors looking to do something different and took a weekend course to learn how to do it. Putting aside how I get paid, I can do whatever I want in medicine with little to no accountability.

Being in the medical errors field has decreased my threshold for shock. A *New England Journal of Medicine* study concluded that as many as 25 percent of all hospitalized patients will experience a preventable medical error of some kind. Almost everyone I talk to has a story about a friend or family member who was hurt, disfigured, or killed by medical mistake. Even me.

My research partner, Peter Pronovost, lost his father due to a medical error when Peter was in medical school. My medical partner, Dr. Patrick O'Kolo, lost his younger sister due to a medical error. My best friend's mom had her breast removed unnecessarily because she was mistakenly told she had stage-three breast cancer. After her procedure, her doctors told her the original report had a mistake—she had only had stage one and hadn't needed a breast removal after all. My grandfather died at age sixty from a condition called urosepsis, a preventable infection following a surgery he didn't even need. My brother has a wide scar on his back from his stitches popping open after a skin mole was removed; he thinks it was unavoidable bad luck, but I can tell the surgeon used stitches too weak to hold the skin together. My cousin worked with a cardiac surgeon and witnessed countless deaths from an impaired physician. I myself was misdiagnosed with a knee problem in medical school.

Listening to Peter and many friends who have similar stories, I realize that these patients suffered not just from their botched treatments but from the knowledge that their misfortune need never have happened. For them, talking about medical mistakes is part of their healing. But our system wants to sweep them under the rug and keep them quiet. I sometimes hear egregious stories from people who preface their accounts with, "Please keep this just between you and me, because I signed a waiver saying that I would never talk about this." When a doctor or hospital does harm a patient, this settlement offer from the hospital often contains a confidentiality clause (a.k.a. "a gag rule"). In fact, in any case of gross neglect, hospital lawyers will aggressively pursue victims or their surviving family to settle out of court quickly in order to stem off a malpractice suit—provided they agree never to speak about what happened, even if one has been disfigured, maimed, or killed.

In order to get a handle on the widespread epidemic of medical mistakes, we need more conversation about them, not less.

There are bad doctors and impaired doctors, but the problem of doctors making repeated avoidable mistakes is a management problem.

Every health services researcher knows errors are common. Medical mistakes are not only far more common than they should be—they are a devastating cost burden on our healthcare system.

Patients under his care suffered because of these communication breakdowns. All this renegade needed was someone higher up the food chain—somebody with authority over his career—to take him aside and tell him to correct his attitude toward his coworkers. That never happened. He continued to terrorize his staff to the detriment of his patients. How can we ensure accountability across the field of healthcare? In principle, most doctors and most hospital administrators agree that accountability is a good thing. But when it comes to being accountable themselves, they are often less enthusiastic. This is only human nature. Taking the extra effort to follow procedures meticulously or keep records of our performance can seem burdensome. And reducing your own accountability can protect your reputation and cover up sins. You are freer to do what you want without having to bother about how other people will react. But a lack of accountability can alienate those who serve and fuel distrust. Moreover, knowing your accountable improves your performance.

Medicine is an institution as old as humanity. Its traditions are as hierarchical as those of the royals. And for centuries, doctors have enhanced their authority with mystery, keeping the workings of their profession opaque. But I am convinced that the new generation of doctors is poised to usher in a revolution of transparency, open-mindedness, and honesty. This generational shift may be just what is needed for medicine to end the secrecy that has historically permeated our profession. With younger doctors taking the lead, the culture is ripe for transformation if we can capitalize on this moment and push for reform from within.

My Response: Accountability is a by-product of AUTHORITY!

I showcased so many of Dr. Makary's quotes because they mirror so well what I have been trying to present to any interested persons, decision makers, and non-decision makers about what is missing, and has always been missing in our healthcare delivery system. The major difference between Dr. Makary's message and mine is that he sees the PROBLEM, while I see both the PROBLEM and the SOLUTION.

Hopefully, Dr. Makary is right, and the "culture" within the medical profession and the hospital administration profession is changing and becoming more receptive to considering fundamental change. Unfortunately, I am not as optimistic. I see no evidence of a desire, or even recognition of a need, to fundamentally change the direction of current efforts, anywhere in the quality of healthcare experts' literature.

"Sue or forget it," and the response it receives from within the quality of healthcare army, if and when coupled with Dr. Makary's well-received *Unaccountable* and its quest for fundamental change, should indicate whether the components of our current healthcare delivery system are truly ready, willing, and able to confront these issues openly and in a meaningful manner.

Doctors Gawande, Makary, and Wachter are at the cutting-edge of the current efforts to make our healthcare delivery system far safer. Time will tell if I will be invited to come under their big tent and contribute to their efforts.

Doctor, Your Patient Will See You Now by Steven Z. Kussin, MD.

Dr. Kussin's book is interesting, particularly for those who decide to take the time to learn as much as possible regarding methods for greater protection when, not if, they or a loved one needs to be hospitalized. Readers need to be prepared, because reading Dr. Kussin's book is a bit like drinking out of a fire hose. This board-certified gastroenterologist was forced to retire from active practice due to an accident not of his own making; therefore, the prospective he provides is both as a caregiver and a care receiver.

Dr. Robert Wachter takes such a prominent role in this, or any other book about the efforts to improve the quality of healthcare because he is a spokesperson for several of the leading components of that collective effort. Also, in this particular reference Dr. Wachter is credited with the creation of what some call the newest medical specialty, Hospitalists.

Hospitalist describe themselves

"Hospitalist" is a relatively recent (first coined in the mid-1990s and more increasing common in the past decade) term for physicians who specialize in the care of patients while they are in the hospital. I will first give a description of this newer form of doctor care, and then quote from Dr. Kussin's rather lengthy contrarian viewpoint.

The hospitalist movement came about due to many factors, which include:

- convenience,
- efficiency,
- financial strain on patients' primary care doctors,
- patient safety,
- cost-effectiveness for hospitals, and
- the need for more specialized and coordinated care for hospitalized patients.

Most hospitalists are board certified internal medicine physicians who have undergone the same training as other internal medicine doctors, including medical school residency training, and board certification examination. The only difference is that hospitalists have chosen not to practice in a traditional outpatient model of internal medicine. Some hospitalists are family practice doctors or medical subspecialists who have opted to do hospitalist work. This can include intensive care specialists, pulmonologists, nephrologists, and other subspecialists.

There are many advantages to using hospitalists in the care of hospitalized patients. One advantage is their added expertise coming from caring for complicated hospitalized patients on a daily basis. They are also more available most of the day in the hospital to meet with family members, able to follow up on tests, answer nurses' questions, and simply deal with problems that may arise. In many instances, hospitalists see a patient more than once a day to assure that care is going according to plan, and explain test findings to patients and family members.

Hospitalists coordinate the care of inpatients, serving as "captain of the ship." They organize the communication between different doctors caring for a patient, and serve as the point of contact for other clinicians for questions, updates, and delineating a comprehensive plan of care. The hospitalist is the main physician for family members to contact for updates on a loved one.

Similarly, because hospitalists are on site at the hospital most of the time, they are able to track test results and order necessary follow-up tests promptly. This is in contrast to the traditional setting where the patient's primary doctor may come to the hospital the next day and take the next necessary follow-up steps at that time.

Because their workplace is the hospital, hospitalists are often more familiar with hospital policies and activities. Many are involved in various hospital committees, and assist in improving important areas such as patient safety, medical error reduction, effective communication between physicians and staff, and cost-effective patient care.

A disadvantage of having a hospitalist take care of you as an inpatient is that he or she may not know your detailed medical history as well as your primary physician. Another potential problem is that your primary care doctor may not have immediate access to the details of your hospitalization care (tests, procedures, results, medications, medical plan of action, etc.). These problems are dealt with to a degree by communication between the primary care doctor and the hospitalist, which ideally takes place at least twice during a hospitalization: at least upon admission and again prior to discharge from the hospital.

The "continuity of care" provided by hospitalists is often described as a clear advantage for better communication and patient comfort.

Dr. Kussin's description of hospitalist:

> Emergencies get you into a hospital. Being in a hospital itself constitutes a state of emergency. Given the intensity of the experience and the consequences of error, this is no time to experiment with the doctors who call themselves hospitalists.
>
> A medical phenomenon, the hospitalist movement is only eleven years old, but is now 30,000 doctors strong. A hospitalist is defined as a physician whose primary duty is the care of hospitalized patients. The hospitalist assumes care of the patient from admission to discharge.
>
> "Continuity of care" is a defining attribute of primary care and a core element of the Institute of Medicine definition of primary care. Continuity is generally recognized to have three dimensions—continuity in information, continuity in management, and continuity in the patient-physician relationship. The dry clay of cost-saving is the soil in which the hospitalist movement was planted. But even the thin sustenance of "dollars saved" is a doubtful proposition.
>
> Hospitalists do not represent a medical specialty. It is not a body of specialized clinical knowledge, nor is it characterized by unique technical skills. There is no specialty licensure, accreditation or state boards, qualifying examinations, or minimum requirements. There are no core undergraduate courses or residencies. Fellowship programs are few and optional. There are no acknowledged standards for mentorship. There is no consistent data on their comparative effectiveness when compared with your own doctor. Membership in the Society of Hospital Medicine, their professional organization, represents only a fraction of its practitioners.

The heterogeneous patient population in hospitals is ill-matched with hospitalists who do not have the skills appropriate for their care. This mismatch of skills is striking and dangerous. Doctors who specialize in internal medicine comprise most of those who identify themselves as hospitalists (85 percent of the total). They are performing duties in areas they are ill-trained to supervise—geriatrics, orthopedics, neurology, and pre-and postoperative care. According to one source, a third of patients require tasks that hospitalists are unfit to handle. The growth in care of surgical patients by medicine physicians raises the issue of appropriate training.

Hospitalists become the least bad performers we learned about in chapter one. And it's all about the money. No medical benefit was demonstrated. Yet, you will find hospitalists in 85 percent of hospitals with 200 or more beds. The acknowledged impetus for the movement and the continued rationale for its existence are monetary—getting you out of the hospital and off its books even faster.

The secondary goal of the hospitalist movement bows to your own doctor, who manages and values his schedule more than he does your care. Bluntly, a hospitalist's job is to decrease not only your length of stay in the hospital but the amount of time your own doctor devotes to your care. But this, one of your most important life choices, is undermined when you're placed in the care of a hospitalist at a time when chance should play no role in your care. Your primary doctor doesn't want to provide services while you are in the hospital; the hospitalist avoids providing services after you've left it. We will see that this line of separation is really a chasm—one into which a majority of patients fall and a great number are subsequently damaged.

Hospitalists are actually primary care doctors who belong in community offices. Instead, the collapsing primary care system, which is now in crisis in part due to their absence, dumps you in the hospital, but ironically increasing the perceived need for even more hospitalists. It's a vicious cycle in which hospitals and doctors scramble to avoid the only obligation that they should never transfer. Continuity of care is a basic tenet of primary care.

Hospitalists bring no special skills, cognitive or procedural, to your bedside aside from their purported, but never proven, superior availability and affordability. Only 50 percent of hospitalists provide care on weekends and off hours. Your hospitalists may work with a clear conflict of interest if his salary, bonus, or income withholds are affected by the speed of your discharge. If so, he is disqualified from your care.

There is no consistent body of evidence demonstrating that hospitalists provide superiority of care over a patient's own physician. You are giving up a lot to gain little or nothing. The bar is set very low for hospitalists. "Non-inferiority" is their benchmark. Yes, "non-inferiority" is the new "better."

While you are in the hospital, your care should be seamless. Under hospitalists there are two euphemistically titled "transition zones" that occur on admission to and discharge from the hospital. These are the breaches into which quality of care can come to grief, but they typically aren't taken into account in quality of care studies. They occur before you are admitted and continue after you've left the hospital. These black holes in the medical literature are the true indicators of the deficiency in the system. The quality of your care decreases and the chance for a fatal error increases simultaneously the moment your doctor relinquishes your care to a hospitalist.

Inadequate communication is responsible for 50 percent of all medication errors. Most of those occur almost immediately when you step through the hospital door. Error is a leading cause of affordable harm suffered by patients, resulting in significantly increase morbidity, prolonged length of stay in hospital, and increased mortality. Medication error occurs most commonly at the interfaces of care. Twenty-five percent of those errors are due to an inadequate medical history and the failure to review your prior medical records.

The interregnum that occurs between your departure from the hospital and your return to your doctor's office is even more prone to serious error. At minimum, your family doctor will need a discharge summary, your physical findings, the results of your testing, and changes in your medication, as well as the reasons for these alterations.

The results of the test you endured, took risk in having, and for which you will be unsparingly billed or incorrectly listed are missing 29 percent of the time. It was shown in 2010 that in the rush to get you out, you, while dusting yourself off at the curb, will still have 40 percent of your test results pending. Forty-three percent of these will show abnormalities; 10 percent of these will be significantly enough to require action; 60 percent of the hospitalists who ordered them are, and will forever be, unaware of them. One to two percent of these abnormalities are so dramatic that they would lead to a change in your diagnosis or therapy. Finally, the fact that fewer than half of the primary care doctors were contacted during a patient's hospitalization or informed of a patient's discharge is indicative of the degree to which primary care physicians are ignored, isolated, and marginalized by the hospitalist system. These facts come from a study of 2,644 patients who were discharged from two Boston hospitals. In another survey of over 900 primary care doctors performed in 2009, the investigators noted, more than half reported not receiving a discharge summary within two weeks, and almost one-quarter did not have any knowledge that their patients had been admitted at all.

My Response: Compare and Contrast the Yin and Yang of "Hospitalists."

Those conflicting views of the newest "kids" on the medical profession's block provide much food for thought, particularly the next time someone who reads this is forced to enter a hospital as a patient. I have a couple of additional thoughts to add to the above mix.

For the past several years when I've had occasions to talk with anyone, the person or a loved one, who has spent considerable time as a patient in a hospital, and where their medical problem required several different practitioners, usually of different specialties, I have asked, "Who was the captain of the ship?"

Consistently, their answer was, "We don't know."

Captain of the Ship

Patients hospitalized with questionable primary-cause medical conditions that require multiple doctors, typically of different specialties, have a right to know who is the captain of their ship at all times; and that label of responsibility should be clearly documented in their medical record. In addition, circumstances may require that label of responsibility to be transferred from the first captain to another doctor. But that, too, should be clearly documented on the patient's medical record. I suspect that the all-important designation of responsibility would be difficult, if not impossible, to find in the majority of patient care cases requiring such. Another point Dr. Kussin neglected to mention came as a small shock to me when I was first told of its probability. Apparently in many, if not most, patient care cases involving hospitalists, the patient may be cared for by a team of rotating hospitalists, and in those cases patient care continuity is wishful thinking.

In addition, I am very curious as to the response Dr. Kussin's book has received, if any, from the Patient Centeredness aficionados. It appeared to me that his book has their best interests in mind; and with the current rate of needless hospital deaths, patients need all of the friends they can get.

Dr. Kussin's book is a very interesting read, particularly for those with a great interest in our current healthcare delivery system, its many problems, and how they might better arm themselves for the next time there is a need for hospital care within their family.

Highest Duty: My Search for What Really Matters by Captain Chesley "Sully" Sullenberger

I was first led to read Sully Sullenberger's book, *Highest Duty,* about his "search for what really matters" because of my affinity for stories about flying. However, I was compelled to include Sully's book in the "Sue or forget it" section of this book due to his collaboration with Dr. Charles Denham, Dennis Quaid, and John Nance as they seek to create a new federal bureaucracy in our healthcare system that would mirror the National Transportation Safety Board.

Dr. Lucian Leape is credited with being the first quality of healthcare expert to push for the inclusion into our healthcare delivery system of many of the safety features that have made our commercial aviation industry so successfully safe. Unfortunately, I have always found the efforts by Dr. Leape, and all others who joined him in that quest, to introduce safety measures from the commercial aviation industry, of trying to do something they did not fully understand. I've always found their concept to be admirable, but their effort is misdirected. I believe that Sully's book *Highest Duty* can help illustrate why commercial aviation is so much safer than patient care in our nation's hospitals.

Sully's quotes: Note: I have found contact with Sully, due to his current national persona, to be impossible, therefore I can only hope that he does not take offense to the following collection of insightful quotes that I feel clearly mesh with the intent of Find The Black Box.

"One thing that has always helped to make the airline industry strong and safe is the concept that pilots call 'captain's authority.' What that means is we have a measure of autonomy—the ability to make an independent, professional judgment within the framework of professional standards."

"With *authority* comes great responsibility."

"Greg Feith, the lead investigator with the National Transportation Safety Board, had told her [Sully's daughter] that her dad's focus would have been on landing the plane. The investigator's words had been somewhat reassuring to her. But in the thirteen years since, she was unable to fully embrace them, because the investigator had never been in a cockpit of a plane in great distress. How could he know what a pilot was truly thinking in such a horrible moment?"

"*Integrity* means doing the right thing even when it's not convenient. Integrity is the core of my profession. I am trained to be intolerant of anything less than the highest standards of my profession."

My Response: I, like everyone else in the nation, have the greatest respect for Sully Sullenberger and his ability to save so many lives, including his own.

But well-deserved adulation should take place within proper context. Throughout my military career, I flew with many outstanding pilots while on active duty and in the reserves, and in two state national guards. Plus, there is a very large number of equally qualified commercial pilots who would have responded in exactly the same way as Sully did, because he simply had no other option than the Hudson River. Any attempt to land on a hard surface runway would have required lowering the landing gear, and that process would have denied him the ability to reach the nearest airport runway at Teterboro in New Jersey. Sully did exactly what he had been training himself to do for many years, just like so many highly qualified surgeons in our nation's healthcare system. (I am sure Sully would agree with me on this point.)

Far more important to me regarding Sully's story are the attempts by Dr. Leape and others to incorporate airline safety measures into our healthcare system, and why I believe those attempts have thus far created negligible improvements throughout that system, and their resultant failure supports the major premise of "Sue or forget it."

"With authority comes great responsibility." Sully's words clearly speak the truth. Meaningful authority is almost impossible to be found within the daily activities of our healthcare delivery system anywhere in this nation. Without an organizational structure, there can be no authority, or delegated authority, that can be applied through responsibility in order to create meaningful accountability.

Sully's entire flying career was spent in two "systems" (the US Air Force and commercial aviation), which both possessed *organizational structure, authority,* and *delegated authority*—indispensable ingredients that apparently Dr. Leape, and too many other quality of healthcare experts, have never recognized! Sully became a check pilot ONLY because his airline could *delegate authority* to him. I became Wing Headquarters Squadron commander at age twenty-three for the same reason.

Healthcare in America will always remain "problematic" until and unless federal and state decision makers recognize the absolute necessity and thus-far absence of those essential ingredients for effective and efficient functioning of any so-called "system."

I have included these book critiques because I believe they, individually and collectively, demonstrate the absence of organizational structure and authority, and the failure by the quality of healthcare experts to *recognize* their absence. Experts on high can continue to write standards and safety measures until the end of time, but unless they recognize the absolute necessity of having an organizational structure with CLEARLY DEFINED points of authority, responsibility, and accountability, we will continue to periodically estimate the current carnage of needless hospital deaths.

"Integrity means doing the right thing even when it's not convenient." I find it incompatible to relate the word integrity to a medical profession that would create the Litigation Center. Sadly, integrity had been replaced by "Sue or forget it" long ago within the "core" of our medical profession. Every time doctors plead for more medical malpractice tort reform, they are simultaneously telling the public: "We will continue to leave you with 'Sue or forget it,' while tipping the scales of justice more and more in our favor in every way we can." Also . . .

If "LOSER PAYS" is attached to medical malpractice tort reform by any state governor and legislature, this will basically entail LEGAL "RAPE" of any person harmed by a doctor!

But back to a kinship I feel between Sully and me . . . .

Sully and I share a similar misgiving regarding our past military life. We were both trained in combat aircraft, but fortunately never faced an enemy. Naturally we both were left to wonder, "Would I have performed the way I like to think I would have performed?" There can never be a definitive answer.

My South Korea-Japan unit island-hopped our WWII planes back across the Pacific in early 1955 to our new base, Eglin #9, Hulbert AFB, Florida. That summer we transitioned into jet engine medium bombers, and I found myself flying at 50,000 ft., where the blue turns black, on the edge of space.

During my first flight at that level, my pilot and I were able to circle the stalk of a Texas thunderstorm while looking up to its anvil-shaped top, probably at 80–85,000 ft. They called that pushing the envelope; and for a twenty-two-year-old, it was as close to heaven as I have been thus far.

On one clear winter night flight at that level out of Blytheville AFB, I could turn my head from right to left and identify the lights of St. Louis, Kansas City, Topeka, Wichita, Tulsa, and the glow of Oklahoma City. As we turned to return home, Milwaukee and Chicago appeared to be connected by a row of streetlights. Little did I know then that I would spend three years of my life in Milwaukee, beginning seven years later, in 1963.

On Saturday, October 28, 1962, I was awakened at midnight and told to report to our unit at the military ramp at Memphis Municipal Airport at 8:00 a.m. I was back on active duty thanks to the Cuban Crisis. That event reduced my internship from twelve months to ten, and appeared to end my process of seeking acceptance to an oral surgery residency program. Our troop carrier Air Force Reserve Unit had focused most of our training on dropping Army parachute trainees at Fort Benning GA, Fort Bragg NC, and Fort Campbell KY.

If we had invaded Cuba, things would have been quite different for our unit. We would have been the first boots on the ground, and I do mean "we." We would have assault-landed at the missile sites and let the troops out the back ramp. That would have instantly turned me into an untrained infantry officer with only a .45 on my hip. Having spent most of my time in my internship in oral surgery with a surgeon who spent time in WWII Europe in a mash unit, I knew that once on the ground I would need to be able to utilize my surgical expertise, such as it was at that time. I bought a Boy Scout backpack and created an emergency kit so that I could extract teeth as needed, close wounds, and wire jaws together. I could certainly do far more good with that kit than I ever could have with that .45. I kept that backpack for quite a few years, just as a reminder of how a turn of events can redirect one's life.

I was selected for the crew to represent our unit at Homestead AFB, south of Miami, the week after the Crisis ceased to be a crisis. President Kennedy had hoped to honor those units recalled to active duty, but his schedule did not permit that ceremony. After five days of staying close to the phone, we were told to return home. Ours, and similar units, were awarded the Presidential Unit Citation. Air Force Major Rudolph Anderson, a U2 pilot from Greenville, SC, was the only combat fatality during the Cuban Crisis and his memorial was rededicated in Greenville in October 2012.

During my three-year oral and maxillofacial surgery residency at Marquette University and the VA hospital in Milwaukee, Wisconsin, I was also a member of the Wisconsin Air National Guard unit as a navigator. That unit's mission was air-to-air refueling; but it also had its own aero club, and that provided me with the opportunity to obtain my private pilot license (single engine). This led me to another great thrill in flying. I was able to arrange a training mission to Frankfort, Germany, in late June 1965 that just coincidentally matched the schedule for the Second International Association of Oral and Maxillofacial Surgeon Conference in Copenhagen, Denmark.

I had to have been the only American oral surgery resident at that conference, but a greater thrill awaited me at the airport. My crew landed at Copenhagen to pick me up; and while the flight plan was being filed and the plane refueled, I noticed some of our crew across the runway gathered around where a Danish Air Force glider was taking off and landing. I hurried over and got in line. When it became my time, I mentioned that I was a pilot. The Danish lieutenant said, "Get in front." It can't get much better than flying a glider over Copenhagen, Denmark, on a gorgeous summer day. The pilot never touched the controls, and I nailed the landing.

Old soldiers can go on and on, but I hope I have made my case that I am fully qualified to participate in any discussions regarding how to incorporate aviation safety procedures into the efforts to make our healthcare delivery system far better. I can hardly wait for that debate. I just hope it will truly be an open and courteous sharing of qualified viewpoints, focused on issues and not persons, and with only positive intent.

The Checklist Manifesto: How to Get Things Right by Atul Gawande, MD.

Dr. Atul Gawande's world-renowned checklist system and book have been discussed and critiqued earlier, but I wanted to reference his system and book in this collection of notable books on healthcare for a particular reason.

Connecting the dots is the theme of this chapter. I believe it's important to read books not only for what they say, but also for what they don't say. Dr. Gawande and the South Carolina Hospital Association chose to partner in a program to institute Dr. Gawande's checklist into as many operating rooms as possible throughout the state's healthcare delivery system, beginning in early 2011. Important here is the means by which Dr. Gawande and the South Carolina Hospital Association can determine how successful their program has been thus far. Unfortunately, after reading several of the books mentioned in this chapter, one can reasonably anticipate that even making those proven-to-be-beneficial patient-safety methods routinely accepted throughout the current medical culture within our hospitals will, in all likelihood, be very difficult.

What is more likely, the South Carolina Hospital Association will resist describing in detail how they hope to determine the success of this new partnership in patient safety, because they have no clearly defined method to obtain such information—so vital to the very purpose of this partnership and to the citizens of South Carolina.

It is one thing to make a great public announcement about the initiation of their combined efforts to make patient care far safer in South Carolina's hospital operating rooms. How to determine the full patient care benefits of this partnership in safety, and how that means of determination will be provided to the public, is their next important step. Harvard Medical School Department of Anesthesia was able to demonstrate rapid patient care improvement in one year due to the use of seven simple "lines in the sand" throughout their system of nine hospital departments of anesthesia.

Their checklist system, suitable for every rural community hospital, as is Dr. Gawande's checklist system, was initiated thirty years ago.

People familiar with our medical profession's literature over several decades are also familiar with the great periodic public claims of fantastic improvements in patient safety "coming soon" due to some new theoretical system that will "change how doctors provide patient care." Sadly, the needless hospital death rate keeps going in the wrong direction. (Perhaps there is something really important missing in our current healthcare delivery system.) Still, every positive attempt to make patient care safer should be recognized and appreciated, i.e., Gawande and Pronovost checklist systems, because they can and do save patient's lives. The problem is making them become as second nature in their use as those checklists were during my military career six decades ago.

The Company That Solved Health Care by John Torinus, Jr.

Everyone who writes a book searches for a title that will grab a potential reader's eye; and certainly this title, *The Company That Solved Health Care* should arrest our attention. Unfortunately a more accurate title, *The Company That Solved Healthcare For Its Company* would not be nearly as eye-catching.

I've included this book and another book, Regina Herzlinger's *Who Killed Healthcare?* in an effort to make what I consider to be one of the most important initial points to understand about our healthcare system's many problems.

Our healthcare system, as I keep repeating, has two equally important aspects: cost and access, and the healthcare delivery system. The overwhelming national focus on the cost and access aspects of our healthcare system, while leaving the tragedy of the needless hospital death rate continuing to go in the wrong direction almost exclusively in the hands of the quality of healthcare experts, is creating far more harm than good.

Cost and access healthcare change seeks to save money. Healthcare delivery system change can save lives AND money. Still, businesses must confront the constantly rising cost of healthcare for the sake of their companies and their employees.

Over the past several years, I have written some thought papers in an effort to describe what I, as someone with experience from within that system, see as factors contributing to the many problems of that system. This next summary is a brief thought paper I wrote just before I came across Mr. Torinus's book.

"What's Really Wrong with Healthcare? The Lament of a Healthcare Heretic" by Dr. Ira Williams

What's really wrong with healthcare? Fundamentally and systematically speaking, almost everything. American healthcare remains, by far, the best in the world (in spite of the WHO skewed ranking), only because so many highly qualified practitioners are able to overcome the enormous deficiencies created by that "system's" complete lack of any systematic characteristics. The easiest way to describe what is wrong with healthcare is to describe several of its problems in random order, with no attempt to rank those problems as worst, or least problematic. What's really wrong with healthcare is their cumulative effect.

Problem: Wrong Model. What was the *model* used to create the foundational base that our current healthcare system rests upon? The nation that allowed men to walk on the moon and return safely also allowed one of its most critically important components (healthcare) to evolve like a weed patch, with NO master gardener.

Doctors ruled the healthcare delivery system with scant and ineffectual outside intrusion. All states (some even prior to statehood) recognized their regulatory responsibility to their citizenry only long enough to individually create state medical examining boards over 100 years ago and they then turned their attention elsewhere.

The era of modern medicine began post-WWII and that *might* have been an ideal time to recognize the need for a properly organized healthcare delivery system. Unfortunately, most leaders and decision makers of that time in our history were survivors of two world wars and the Great Depression, and suddenly then confronted by the shock of the Korean War and its oppressive appendage, the Cold War. The time was right, but the necessary creators were nonexistent. The complete absence of any deep consideration ever being given to how an organizational structure should (must) be constructed within the framework of our form of federal/state governmental responsibility deserves recognition.

Problem: Absence of an Organizational Structure. Even with the absence of a working model for the constant remodeling of healthcare delivery, the three major components of our healthcare system (organized medicine, federal government, and state governments) persisted in creating "change" within their purview of that system, with little recognition of the other components. In essence, each major component did their thing while all three were playing in the same sandbox.

Try effectively using a large, multi-component, technologically laden system necessary for the well being of all citizens that is completely lacking in a recognizable organizational structure. We have been doing that for far too long, and the results are constant chaos and diminishing effectiveness, resulting in the enormous loss of lives unnecessarily.

However, it seems that saying that our healthcare system lacks an organizational structure has less impact than saying the Chicago Cubs will not win the World Series again this year, thereby reinforcing the understanding that it is hard to prove a negative. Why should anyone care that our healthcare system has always lacked an organizational structure? Armed services (Army, Navy, Air Force) and large, multi-factory companies demonstrate the need and benefit of organizational structure as containing clearly defined points of *authority, responsibility,* and *accountability* at established levels throughout their structures. A detailed comparison of our current healthcare system with the organizational structure of the Air Force would rapidly illustrate the disastrous results inherent in the absence of effective agents of authority and accountability at every level. Having personal experience in specific instances demanding the effective use of authority and accountability in both the Air Force and our healthcare system, I have participated in the benefits of the former and the degradation of the latter.

Problem: Absence of Authority and Accountability. Authority (the buck stops here) *must* be present, accepted as such, and constantly functioning for accountability to contribute to the effectiveness of any system. There is a simple, but sad, test one might utilize to demonstrate the absence of authority and accountability in our healthcare system. Needless hospital deaths (never events) have been a recognized tragedy throughout our nation's hospitals for over twenty years. Beginning immediately after the fact, track and document how any state healthcare delivery system responds to such an event and (sadly) visualize the enormous failure of every state governor and legislature, past and present. One can only ask, "Does anybody care?"

Every state created a medical state board of examiners with the purpose to "regulate" the practice of medicine. Most, if not all, states have also created at least one agency with some semblance of *authority* over hospitals. Yet the results are that our nation's hospitals are the only place in America where an accidental death (never event) receives NO immediate response and review by a source of state authority.

People decry the chaos in our current healthcare system while, at the same time, no one can provide a detailed description of that "system" and identify that system's points of authority, responsibility, and accountability.

Test: America has over forty schools of public health with some dating back to early in the last century. I ask again if any of these schools has even one department head or professor who has taught and written on the twin facts that since state's license doctors to practice medicine and all medical care is local, then each state is responsible to its citizens to establish and support a functional healthcare delivery system.

Even if a perfect system for how to pay for healthcare after the fact suddenly materialized, chaos would continue to reign until and unless every state's responsibility for their healthcare delivery system is recognized and provided for.

About a week after writing this, I came across Mr. Torinus's book, read it and called him. He very kindly spoke with me, and I told him I had written a well-intended critique of his book and would like to send it to him; and he accepted my offer.

The Company that Solved Healthcare: How Serigraph Dramatically Reduced Skyrocketing Costs While Providing Better Care, and How Every Company Can Do the Same by John Torinus, Jr.

My Critique

Any attempt to critique, even with positive intent, *The Company That Solved Healthcare* will likely be viewed as akin to desecrating the grave of Mother Teresa. Still, the very title of the book and its exuberant claim literally shouts for critical review.

The first point that should be made is that the total body of positive methods of confronting the constantly rising cost of how to pay for healthcare far outweighs the distorted claim within the title. The many problems of our nation's healthcare system have NOT been "solved" by John Torinus, Jr., and his dynamic band of supporters. Furthermore, *The Company That Solved Healthcare* fails to recognize one of, if not the most important, failure of our current healthcare system. That said, this critique with positive intent will continue.

First, about the blurbs: Praise for *The Company That Solved Healthcare*:

Paul O'Neill, former CEO of Alcoa and secretary of the Treasury, said, "The healthcare industry is badly in need of new business models and systems thinking."

Probably the best point to begin in attempting to describe the inherent failure(s) of our healthcare system is to recognize the fact that there has *never been* an original "model" upon which our current healthcare system was allowed to be formed and periodically modified. Our healthcare system has evolved like a weed patch, with no master gardener.

Greg Scandlen, editor, *Consumer Power Report* said, "This book describes the real-world revolution that is transforming healthcare into a cost-efficient, accountable system through empowering consumers."

Mr. Torinus has NOT solved healthcare; there is NO real-world revolution transforming any state's healthcare delivery system; and empowering consumers is NOT going to make healthcare in America all that we wish it to be. Mr. Torinus's wonderful cost-containing efforts have NOT changed the structural deficiencies within our current healthcare system. Those who want proof need to compare the estimated annual rate of needless hospital deaths in 1990 to the current estimated annual rate and discover that there are far more *never events* now than two decades ago, and no one is asking Why?

The purpose of these two examples of the multitude of laudatory expressions gathered to rightfully praise Mr. Torinus's status as a "national treasure" [Regina E. Herzlinger] are offered to illustrate what Mr. Torinus, his army of supporters, and through his many achievements have failed to recognize, but more on that later.

Selected Quotes: from the Introduction, "Real Reform of Healthcare Still To Come"

"This book is a story of the development of a business model that brings sanity back to the economic side of medicine."

"The root cause of the problem has been ineffective cost management."

"If our political leaders had listened to the pioneers in healthcare delivery, the huge bill for universal coverage could have been paid for with savings from better business models."

My Response: There are two distinctly different aspects of our healthcare system: cost and access, or how to pay for healthcare after the fact, and the healthcare delivery system. Both aspects are, and have always been, severely flawed, but each aspect for different reasons. Even if a solution for the cost and access aspect of healthcare was suddenly, magically found, the healthcare delivery system would remain unorganized and dysfunctional.

Those "pioneers in healthcare delivery" that Mr. Torinus refers to are currently leading the efforts to improve the quality of healthcare in the wrong direction, and a thorough consideration of *all* of the facts supports that contention. Even more troubling should be the recognition that probably most quality of healthcare experts desire, and are working toward, complete control of all aspects of healthcare by the federal government (per their literature).

"That means identifying and promoting what Serigraph calls "centers of value," where value means the best combination of service, quality, and price."

Quality is a word copiously used in almost every discussion regarding the problems of healthcare, yet a specific description of the "quality," both acceptable and unacceptable, of the most common medical forms of patient care can never be determined within the medical community. One must read great quantities of the medical literature regarding the quality of patient care in order to recognize how nebulous the ability is to speak in specifics regarding the true "quality" of healthcare.

Also, there is, and has always been, a value to healthcare in America, because we were founded upon a free enterprise system whereby medical care was inherently a consumer product, i.e., a house, a car, or a loaf of bread. The argument, "Is healthcare a right or a privilege?" is one with seemingly no clear answer thus far. Give the federal government sufficient time, and they will decide the issue; however, the result may not be in the best interests of most people.

"Ideally, Robin should have been able to view comparative quality as well." Those who believe that "data on healthcare" is going to miraculously improve the quality of healthcare at some time in the future are waiting for the Titanic to dock in NYC. A critique does not permit sufficient time and space to demonstrate how and why the current efforts to improve the quality of healthcare lack the fundamental requirement necessary to make those efforts beneficial. I am prepared to accept any challenge to that claim, provided I am given sufficient time and courtesy.

"It has been a long tenet of Serigraph to 'demanage'—to put decision making into the hands of the people doing the actual work in what we call natural work units." In essence, Serigraph delegates authority at various levels within their organizational structure. Such a positive attribute for efficient activity within any system is sorely lacking in our healthcare system and will be discussed in more detail later.

Price not related to quality? There's that Q-word again. Rarely have so many learned individuals talked more and understood less than is known and *understood* about the quality of healthcare, particularly in cases of questionable patient care. You don't understand a subject that you cannot clearly describe and define, and no one involved in the quality of healthcare issues can provide a clear description and a clear definition of the quality of healthcare, particularly in those cases where such is most needed, i.e., when a patient has been medically harmed.

"And we are finding potential savings everywhere in the broken delivery system." Quite possibly the most universally accepted mistakes in the efforts to improve our healthcare system is the failure to *completely separate* and *isolate one from the other*—cost and access (how to pay for healthcare after the fact) from the healthcare delivery system. People sick or injured enter the healthcare delivery system, and that is where the quality of healthcare and patient care accountability must be confronted. Any inclusion of cost and access issues into considerations for how to improve the healthcare delivery system will completely disrupt those efforts. Yet the first and foremost issue regarding our healthcare problems is how to pay for it. Both aspects of that system are equally important, and each aspect in its own way is equally "broken." Their individual complexities demand that they each be considered and dealt with separately. I have come to understand how difficult this concept is to grasp, but such separation actually makes understanding of each less confusing.

"The medical side of healthcare is often brilliant (and also not so brilliant). There is spectacular innovation and intimate caregiving. That is not where the problem lies, though there is much room for improvement on quality, including elimination of errors."

I have written two books largely dealing with the problems within the "medical side of healthcare," and this oversimplification of one of the major causes of the constantly rising cost of healthcare trivializes the dark side of healthcare. True transformation of healthcare can only occur if and when we can better deal with "questionable" patient care.

"Doctors know who the good doctors are." Doctors also know who the bad doctors are, BUT THEY DON'T TALK ABOUT THOSE. Wisconsin created their medical examining board in 1897 with a major part of their mission statement being the regulation of medical practitioners; and, 115 years later, what does the WMEB have to show for its efforts? Every state's medical board has been as effective as the UN has been in stopping genocide in Darfur. WMEB was delegated authority and has never developed a mechanism necessary to fulfill their responsibility. More importantly, there are clearly evident reasons why they have failed, as has every other state medical board in identifying the "bad doctors" from the "good doctors." Those who really want to cut the cost of healthcare must find a way to better identify problem practitioners. The medical profession has never been able to do so.

(Chapter 9) Quality Ratings *Elusive,* But Essential: BOY! You said a mouth full there! First, just try to identify all the agencies and organizations with a Q in their acronym that are active in issues involving the quality of healthcare. Next, try to determine if we are any closer to being able to clearly describe the quality of patient care, particularly when questions of care arise, and more particularly at a few hospitals near you.

(Chapter 11) Silver Bullet for Better Value: Lean Disciplines That Transform: Like Chapter 9, the issues regarding the delivery of healthcare contained here are the subject of books and years of research. Yet the key element is missing thus far in the healthcare literature.

"What's really needed is a new *business* model." What is really needed is a new *healthcare delivery model.* ObamaCare, RomneyCare and even ClintonCare are/were attempts to save money in healthcare. A new healthcare delivery system, properly structured, would save *lives and money.*

Summary: My, at times, harsh critique has no intent to "rain on your parade." I genuinely applaud your outstanding accomplishments in healthcare cost containment, as well as all of the other similar efforts throughout the nation. South Carolina Business Coalition on Health held an all-day meeting here in Greenville on May 8, 2012, and Dr. Zastrow was one of several presenters in the morning half of that program. The afternoon was devoted to multiple breakout sessions. I attended the two sessions focused on South Carolina collaboration with IHI in their Triple Aim endeavor.

I left that program galvanized by two separate thoughts: First, the many positive efforts to reduce the cost of healthcare in places like Wisconsin, Cincinnati, St Louis, etc. But the more disturbing thought focused on all that was never mentioned. Thought papers on my web site (healhc.com) were all written in the next two days following that SCBCH meeting.

My web site, video, and thought papers provide considerable insight into my great concern that NO ONE in or outside the healthcare system appears to recognize the state's (every state's) responsibility for their healthcare delivery system. They remain clueless.

Mr. Torinus, I can speak in great detail regarding:

- Why and how every state's healthcare delivery system is broken.
- How to completely reorganize state healthcare delivery systems.
- Why efforts by IOM, AHRQ, IHI, NQF, NPSF, etc., are unable to ever provide the benefits to the quality of healthcare they claim.

Dr. Robert Wachter and I had a brief, but very telling conversation here in Greenville in September 2010. The public should know the details of that conversation and subsequent events because there is much the public is not being told about the efforts to improve the quality of healthcare in America.

I want to share with you an email exchange between Dr. Wachter and me the Monday following our brief meeting.

On October 4, 2010, at 8:47 a.m., Dr. Ira Williams wrote:

> Dr Wachter,
>
> I thoroughly enjoyed your presentation and our brief conversation. I also read *Balancing "No Blame"* and I feel I now have a far more clear understanding of how our individual approaches to making healthcare safer both differ and benefit each other.
>
> Our healthcare system can never be what it should be until and unless we vastly improve systems errors and practitioner errors. I can provide a system of medial peer review fair to both doctor and patient that will enhance your efforts directed toward the other class of medical errors.
>
> I can also provide a system for getting those patient care improvements into all of our nation's hospitals.

In Balancing "No Blame" you and Dr Pronovost say, "Our goal is simply to promote conversations and meaningful action." Is there room in your big patient safety tent for me?

It is very easy for those who do not know me to judge me in a harsh and negative manner. I hope someday to be considered one of the best friends your profession has ever had. I hope you will consider my offerings in *Misdiagnosed!* from that perspective. I know how and where to make real healthcare patient safety happen. I would love to join you in conversation and meaningful action. We must reverse the twenty-year trend of needless hospital deaths.

Sincerely and respectfully,

Dr. Ira Williams

October 4, 2010 12:54:50 p.m. EDT

Thanks, Dr. Williams. I read your book on the way home. You make some important points, and I agree that peer review is a critical, and mostly neglected, component of patient safety.

I'll keep you in mind for appropriate opportunities, but don't have any right now.

Best regards.
—Bob

I have never heard from Dr. Wachter since.

Mr. Torinus, I do not understand why every door to discussions regarding how to improve the quality of healthcare are closed to me. I know how to really change healthcare in every hospital and surgery center in our nation. I hope someone will accept my well-intended challenge.

I hope you will visit my web site, read my short video and my thought papers.

I would love to return to Wisconsin and share my expertise with those who are interested in hearing what no one else is talking about.

I look forward to hearing from you.

Sincerely,
Dr. Ira Williams

Mr. Torinus and I spoke again while I was seeking permissions and he graciously consented to my including portions of his book in my book. He also wished me good luck in my pursuit in trying to do for the healthcare delivery system what he and his company have done for their portion of the cost & access aspect of healthcare.

The Creative Destruction of Medicine: How the Digital Revolution Will Create Better Health Care by Eric Topol, MD

Note: Dr. Topol rapidly responded "Yes, and good luck!", to my request for permission.

excerpts: from the Introduction:

In the mid-twentieth century Joseph Schumpeter, the noted Austrian economist, popularize the term "creative destruction" to denote transformation that accompanies radical innovation. In recent years, our world has been "Schumpetered."

There is legitimate worry about adoption of new technologies before they had been adequately vetted and validated, or proven to be cost-effective and ideally cost saving. Ultimately, you will have to decide about the trade-offs of medicine Schumpetered. This book is intended to put you in position to be ready and knowledgeable to make that decision.

Another major deficiency of medicine is the use of experts to make recommendations or "guidelines" for a large proportion of decisions for which no or minimal data exists. These guidelines, typically published in major specialty journals, have a pronounced impact, as they are believed to represent the standard of care, even though they are based on opinion with a paucity of facts. In fact, this should be considered "eminence- based medicine." As we are able to accrue more meaningful data and information on individuals, the hope is that we can override our dependence on such recommendations.

In the meantime, flawed evidence-based medicine of today is being advocated to provide immunity from medical malpractice. In a *New York Times* op-ed, Peter Orszag, formerly the director of the White House Office of Management and Budget, suggested that we could "provide safe harbors for doctors who follow evidence-based guidelines." The 2009 US economic stimulus act promoted comparative effectiveness in medical research and the new Patient-Centered Outcomes Research Institute. Unfortunately, the funding is disproportionate with the relative void of information, and the efforts that are being mounted are tied to population medicine. It's ironic that the new initiative is called "Patient Centered"—if only that were the case.

In 2005 John Ioannidis, now at Stanford University, published the article "Why Most Published Research Findings Are False" in the *Journal PLoS Medicine*, sending chills through the academic medical community. His conclusions are in keeping with what has been reviewed here: (1) the smaller the studies, the less likely the research findings are to be true; (2) the smaller the effect, the less likely the research findings are to be true; (3) the greater the financial and other interest, the less likely the research findings were to be true; (4) the hotter a scientific field (with more scientific teams involved), the less likely the research findings are to be true.

Unlike our legal system, in which a defendant is considered innocent until proven guilty, new scientific or medical evidence has to refute and transcend the "null-hypothesis." In other words, consider the new findings null and void unless you are thoroughly convinced that the evidence is compelling. I coined the term "litter-ature" to denote that too much of the medical literature is littered with misleading and false-positive findings. That there is simply too much literature (and litter- ature) is evidenced by the statistic that only 0.5 percent of the thirty-eight million published papers are cited more than two hundred times by others, and half were never cited. Moreover, when pooled analyses of prior studies are published, many relevant papers are excluded.

One patient had sixty-seven stents placed throughout his coronary arteries and bypass grafts, in the course of twenty- eight coronary angiograms over a ten-year period. This problem of inappropriate use or overuse of medical procedures is a difficult nut to crack. (I know how to crack that nut.)

Electronic Health Records (EHRs) and Health Information Technology (HIT)*(from Chapter 7)*

In 1999 Institute of Medicine published a report *To Err Is Human*, which proclaimed that "at least 44,000 people, and perhaps as many as 98,000 people, die hospitals each year as a result of medical errors that could have been prevented," but which arose because "faulty systems, processes, and conditions" led people either to make mistakes or to fail to prevent them. Medical errors are far more common and serious then had generally been perceived, and certainly far greater than what I had ever estimated. This alarming exposé of medical errors raised awareness of how poorly and chaotically patient data is recorded and how it is notoriously inaccessible—perhaps representing the root cause of the problem.

An alarming *Washington Post* editorial on the subject, "A Medical Enron," declared that "these various errors reflect the arrogance of the medical priesthood" and "thousands will continue to die needlessly with no one held to account." A *New York Times* article on the day the report was released described a possible remedy: the report called for a new Center for Patient Safety and the minimum goal of reducing medical errors by 50 percent in the following five years. There was a surprising omission in the plans, however: the computerization of medical records.

But the next Institute of Medicine (IOM) report on the subject—*Crossing the Quality Chasm: A New Health System for the 21st Century*, published in March 2001—zeroed in on health information technology: "Healthcare organizations, hospitals and physician groups typically operate as separate 'silos,' acting without the benefit of complete information about the patient's condition." "The committee calls for a nationwide infrastructure to support healthcare delivery, consumer health, quality measurement and improvement, public accountability, clinical and health services research and clinical education. This commitment should lead to the elimination of most handwritten clinical data by the end of the decade."

Now a decade later, there is little to show for this shout- out. There is minimal hard evidence for either the reduction of medical errors or the adoption of electronic medical records. In a report in late 2010 in the *New England Journal of Medicine*, ten well-regarded North Carolina hospitals described how, having actively pursued quality improvement measures to reduce errors, they tracked 2,341 admissions between 2002 and 2007 to see whether there was evidence of improvement during that time. The data showed none. There were more than sixty patient injuries per 1,000 patient days both at the beginning and at the end of the study. Roughly two-thirds were deemed preventable. Overall, some form of harm to patients accompanied 25 percent of hospital admissions. In 2011, the journal *Health Affairs* published a special issue, "Still Crossing the Chasm of Quality," with multiple articles on the persistent and serious problems related to medical errors. One group calculated the yearly cost of the errors in the United States was more than 17 billion dollars, another found that the actual number of errors could be ten times greater than the estimates, and an expert in this topic from John's Hopkins, Peter Pronovost, wrote, "For the past decade, healthcare quality has largely sought quick fixes and run from science; the results are evident.

The ultimate solution to this enormous problem is electronic recordkeeping. Of more than 3,000 American hospitals surveyed in 2009, only 1.5 percent had fully electronic health records and health information technology (HIT) systems, and these were largely confined to large teaching hospitals and big cities.

Unbuilding a Tower of Babel

Digitizing the words and files from the hospital chart of the doctor's office notes is the core of the electronic health (or medical) record. Ideally, the EHR, as it is more frequently being referred to, would be a comprehensive file that includes all laboratory data and reports from procedures, operations, diagnostic tests, hospital discharges, and office visits with all physicians and healthcare practitioners. *The remarkable fragmentation of the American healthcare system makes this difficult.* Taken together, we get fragmentation to an exponential level. You might just call it chaos, or a Tower of Babel. The buzzword goal to achieve is "interoperability." "Inoperable" is perhaps the best description of our current, incomparable systems.

In 2009 a group of University of Minnesota researchers followed four years of Medicare data to determine whether EHRs had any improvement in patient safety, and they found minimal evidence of support—such as two infections fewer each a year at an average hospital. They concluded, "Health IT's true value remains uncertain." On the other hand, despite experts' optimism, there is currently no evidence that the use of EHRs reduces diagnostic errors. Just collecting data without processing it into actionable information and providing vital feedback to physicians, nurses, and patients, is not enough. Automating a broken process won't provide the fix.

Doctors with plasticity?

Atherosclerosis, referring to a progressive and degenerative process of artery walls, is typically translated for a lay audience as "hardening of the arteries." We've never needed a similar word to describe the medical community. It came with sclerosis built in. Of all the professions represented on the planet, perhaps none is more resistant to change then physicians. If there were ever a group defined by lacking plasticity, it would first apply to doctors.

My thoughts regarding Dr. Topol's thoughts:

Picture a clear, fall night, and a harvest moon illuminating the countryside. Dr. Topol's book describes the future of medical care appearing as bright as the harvest moon. Unfortunately, our healthcare delivery system has a dark side, like the moon. That side is illustrated by the books of Doctors Makary, Wachter, and Lundberg (the latter two brief reviews follow). They're all speaking and writing about the same healthcare delivery system; they all recognize that system's chaotic inability to function in a reasonable manner; yet none of those authors appear to recognize the absence of, or the need for, an organizational structure, and/or the responsibility of each and every state to provide leadership in that regard.

Dr. Topol's book received well-deserved praise from fifteen eminent sources inside, and five more on the back of the jacket cover, exalting his efforts to communicate what hopefully lies ahead for both care-receivers and caregivers in the not too distant future. Dr. Topol also recognizes the many obstacles that will, regardless of the sense of urgency, delay those promised healthcare advancements.

Where I feel Dr. Topol and I are most aligned is in what I perceive to be a mutual anxiety regarding the overwhelming rush to create "centralized initiatives," i.e., national standards, evidence-based medicine, serious reportable events (reported to whom?), and now patient-centered research, etc.—all of which have positive intent, but are offered to a non-system that lacks the ability to disseminate positive improvements throughout that "system."

Internal Bleeding: The Truth Behind America's Terrifying Epidemic of Medical Mistakes by Robert M. Wachter, MD and Kaveh G. Shojania, MD.

> Excerpt taken from the cover flyleaf:
> *Internal Bleeding* exposes the dark secrets behind the glittering façade of modern medicine. Doctors Robert Wachter and Kaveh Shojania, two of the world's foremost authorities on medical mistakes, shatter the silence to tell the dramatic and compelling stories of real patients betrayed by a system they trusted to save them.
> Robert M Wachter, MD, professor of Medicine at the University of California, San Francisco UC SF is chief of the Medical Service at UCSF Medical Center and founding chair of UCSF's Patient Safety Committee. He was the first elected president of the Society of Hospital Medicine (Hospitalist), and has published 150 scholarly articles on topics ranging from patient safety to the organization of hospital care. He is lead editor of the two major academic series on medical

errors in the US ("Quality Grand Rounds" and AHRQ *WebM&M*) and edits the popular textbook *Hospital Medicine*.

~

Doctors Wachter and Shojania's book *Internal Bleeding* was first published the same year that my book *First, Do No Harm* was released in 2004. Much can be gained by those with significant interest in the problems of our healthcare system by reading their book.

However the focus of my critique of *Internal Bleeding* begins with the subtitle of their book, *The Truth Behind America's Terrifying Epidemic of Medical Mistakes*, and the fundamental differences by which Dr. Wachter and I view our nation's terrifying epidemic of medical mistakes.

Doctors Wachter and Shojania's interpretation of the root cause of this terrifying epidemic is now, and will remain, the by-product of medical malpractice litigation (Sue or forget it); and, therefore, the doctors' major problems in this aspect of patient care is primarily somebody else's fault (a litigious society and greedy attorneys). I continue with the belief that as long as "Sue or forget it" remains, overwhelmingly, the system of choice for the review of questionable patient care, chaos will continue to reign within our healthcare delivery system.

Therefore I wish to make an offer that I hope Dr. Wachter and his AHRQ *WebM&M* program can't refuse. I suggest that Dr. Wachter and I have a face-off regarding America's terrifying epidemic of medical mistakes. He might come armed with a copy of *Internal Bleeding*, and I will come armed with a copy of *First, Do No Harm*.

Hospitals are the only place in America where an accidental death receives no immediate review by a state source of authority. That fact demonstrates that those decision makers who possessed the responsibility to regulate professional activities have failed miserably in their efforts to provide meaningful accountability within their medical communities.

Internal Bleeding had publicly acknowledged the fact that there is *no accountability* within our healthcare system several years before Dr. Makary titled his book *Unaccountable*. Doctors Wachter and Makary give passing acknowledgment that medical peer review is somewhere in their hospital medical staff structure; but neither they, nor any other quality of healthcare expert, can speak with any degree of medical expertise regarding what should be the first stage in the review of questionable patient care.

Medical "authorities" periodically and publicly express the great need for an "open debate," but I am unaware of such debates, structured along the lines of the full meaning of that word, ever taking place. Dr. Donald Palmisano, then AMA president-elect, on a video made for public consumption, voiced such a great need in 2003. I wrote Dr. Palmisano a letter accepting his offer, but he replied there was insufficient time in his busy schedule. But our short, cordial exchange when I flew to Chicago in June 2004 and met him briefly during the AMA National Meeting was much like my similar exchange with Dr Wachter in 2010—it failed to initiate a debate. Dr. Palmisano had previously said open debate could prove to be so beneficial for the public. Only time can tell if Dr. Denham, Sully

Sullenberger, Dennis Quaid, and John Nance are truly serious about their desire for an "open debate" regarding their quest for a new National Healthcare Safety Board.

My "debate card" has many openings. Dr. Wachter controls the lineup of his guests on the AHRQ *WebM&M* program of conversations. However, I think such a debate would best serve the public if recorded before a large, live audience. (One can dream.)

Who Killed Healthcare? America's $2 Trillion Medical Problem– and the Consumer-driven Cure by Regina Herzlinger.

It is impossible, as it should be, for any person to write a serious nonfiction book that doesn't initiate well-intended criticism. However, I have only one major criticism with Professor Herzlinger's book, *Who Killed Healthcare?* My criticism is based upon one of the most important, first understandings that people must recognize regarding all of the problems within our healthcare system—that our nation's healthcare system is comprised of two major aspects: cost and access (how to pay for healthcare after the fact), and the healthcare delivery system, which is a state responsibility (every state).

Professor Herzlinger is highly qualified to participate in any and every discussion regarding how to improve the cost and access aspect of our nation's healthcare dilemma. But as I said earlier, with the utmost courtesy and respect, Professor Herzlinger doesn't know beans about the healthcare delivery system. Yet throughout her book, she attempts to weave the two aspects together; and when that is attempted, it invariably leads to increased confusion.

Medicare, Medicaid, insured, uninsured, uninsurable and all the rest of any potential effort that requires someone to pay for healthcare received is a process that occurs after the healthcare fact. Patients, sick or injured, enter the healthcare delivery system; and, I fear, until and unless we can recognize the great benefit that can be achieved by total isolation of any considerations of either aspect, one from the other, all efforts to affect meaningful healthcare change will continue to be as torturous and unproductive as they have been thus far.

As noted earlier, there are multiple congressional subcommittees in both houses of Congress; and I have long felt, as have so many others, that those leaders, with I assume the best of intentions, have consistently done more harm than good.

Every author has a great desire to obtain blurbs from highly recognized sources and I want to read one specific blurb, obtained by Professor Herzlinger, and acknowledge its author.

> "Regi Herzlinger has brilliantly articulated a better way— embracing the principles of competition and innovation that cause each other sector of our economy to thrive. Discharging American healthcare from the ICU can only happen by putting individual Americans—not politicians and bureaucrats— back in charge of their healthcare decisions. US Senator Tom Coburn, MD (OK)."

[I have tried to gain access to Dr./Senator Coburn without success, but I will continue to try.]

Severed Trust: Why American Medicine Hasn't Been Fixed— and What We Can Do About It by George D. Lundberg, MD

I include Dr. Lundberg's book in this collection of reviews for several reasons, and the *first reason* is *Autopsies*.

> **Selected quotes:**
>
> Studies from autopsies even in the 1990s have shown that a remarkably high percentage of causes of death entered by attending physicians are incorrect. Here is an example in which the self-interest of the providers, hospitals, and physicians takes precedent over the interest of science and patient care. When the American Medical Association talks about quality, what it really means is letting doctors do and order whatever they wish, and thereby letting them make as much money as they can.
>
> There is no better way to study the natural history of disease. But among the most important features of the autopsy is that it's the final and definitive method of monitoring the quality of care given to a seriously ill patient or provided by a medical system. Much can be learned about how a society lives by studying how its members die. The most important reason for autopsy is that, when performed correctly, it provides the ultimate control over the assurance of quality in medicine.
>
> Pathologists were the main quality control people in the practice of medicine for much of my career. Mortality conferences were regular, routine events at every major hospital in the developed world and the United States during the fifties and sixties, when autopsy rates were in the range of 50 to 70 percent. I saw firsthand exactly how much physicians learned about medicine when they studied it from this perspective.

Dr. Lundberg appeared on a CBS *60 Minutes* program and was interviewed by Mike Wallace. That program aired in October 1998 and was repeated in July 2000. Dr. Lundberg stated, "I gave the official AMA position on the autopsy: autopsies are good, and more of them ought to be done." This was a long-standing AMA policy which had been elaborated upon and reaffirmed many times.

[Note: I performed thirty-five autopsies during my six-month Pathology rotation in the second half of 1964, and feel strongly that my responsibility to perform the complete autopsy, select the tissue to be microscopically examined, exam same, and file a complete report identifying the *primary cause* and *secondary or contribution cause(s) of death* greatly contributed to my ability to provide better care once in private practice, in the real world.]

Second reason: Perspective.

Dr. Lundberg's book, published in 2001, while using different words, describes the same, or highly similar, dark side to our nation's healthcare delivery system as Drs. Wachter, Gawande, Kussin, and Makary's books. Meaning: nothing meaningful has changed, or gotten better, (Why Haven't We Gotten Further?) in the past decade, or more, and in spite of enormous effort by an army of quality of healthcare experts.

"In order to fix our broken system of American healthcare . . .," he, like all the others, offers "quick-fix" generalities.

Third reason: Medical Ethics.

Medical ethics has been of special interest to me ever since I first came face-to-face with its absence in the real world of our medical profession in Madison, Wisconsin, shortly after entering private practice. Dr. Lundberg's book provides an excellent opportunity to go to the heart of that matter.

> **Excerpt** (from Dr. Lundberg's book):
> In October 1998 I was in Hong Kong as an invited speaker at an international medical congress. Several hundred researchers were there, representing many countries, languages, cultures, and institutions. As the editor of the *Journal of the American Medical Association*, I was assigned to a panel on medical ethics, specifically the ethics of medical journals. The topic was close to my heart. During my seventeen years as editor of *JAMA*, many of the articles and studies that I published on health and social issues also had ethical overtones.
>
> These included calls for gun controls, seatbelt and motorcycle helmet legislation, curbs on drunken-driving, a total ban on boxing, and challenges to the process of how medical journals work. Some of my positions on these and other issues took me outside the mainstream medical establishment, but all were mediated by ethical considerations.
>
> What I didn't know on the flight back from Hong Kong was that the end of my tenure at *JAMA* was only weeks away. It was a public event, intensely covered by the media at a press conference called by the AMA on Friday, January 15, 1999. The headlines told the story. "Editor Fired for Article on Definition of Sex"; "Science, Sex, and Semantics; The Firing of George Lundberg"; and "AMA Firing Impolitic—Or Just Politics?"
>
> The event that precipitated my parting of the ways with the AMA was related to my decision to publish an unsolicited, peer-reviewed study by researchers at the Kinsey Institute at Indiana University who surveyed college student attitudes about sex. Fifty-nine percent said that they did not consider having oral sex as having "had sex." The article appeared in *JAMA* during the Senate impeachment trial of President Clinton. It was said that I had inappropriately and inexcusably interjected *JAMA* into the middle of a debate that had nothing to do with science

or medicine. Not surprisingly, editors and journalists expressed alarm about what they saw as a challenge to editorial independence.

But Dr. Lundberg's hasty dismissal as editor of *JAMA* is not my focus here. Dr. Catherine DeAngelis became the first woman to become the editor of *JAMA* in 2000. Dr. DeAngelis left as editor in chief of the *JAMA* in June 2011 and returned to John's Hopkins University School of Medicine in Baltimore to develop a Center for Professionalism in Medicine and the Related Professions. "I'm going to return to my academic home," she said, adding that the Center for Professionalism will study the ethics of medicine, nursing, and public health as well as healthcare business and law.

The study of ethics (her words) "might (should) begin with, what does AMA think about medical ethics?"

2003 AMA Principles of Medical Ethics

> Principle II. A physician shall uphold the standards of professionalism, be honest in all professional interactions, and strive to report physicians deficient in character or competence, or engaging in fraud or deception, to appropriate entities.

1980 AMA Principles of Medical Ethics:

> 2. A. physician shall deal honestly with patients and colleagues and strive to *expose* those physicians deficient in character or competence, or who engage in fraud.

Taken a step further, what is a medical ethicist?

Dr. Katrina Bramstedt answered:

> A medical ethicist is also sometimes called a clinical ethicist or bioethicist. These are healthcare professionals with either a PhD or MD/DO and advanced fellowship training who specialized in helping patients, families, and medical teams solve medical ethics dilemmas. They also commonly work with medical teams who use high-tech therapies such as organ transplantation and deep brain stimulation.
>
> A medical ethicist is not the same as an ethics committee. An ethics committee is a group of hospital volunteers from a variety of backgrounds (e.g., social work, nursing, psychology, pastoral care, medicine) who meet usually monthly to work on ethical problems/issues in the hospital setting. The members generally have very basic ethics training (e.g., a few seminars, workshops). Sometimes a professional medical ethicist is a member of an ethics committee but not always. Generally, large, academic medical centers employ professional medical ethicist;

whereas community hospitals rely solely on their ethics committee for handling ethical dilemmas. Professional ethicists are also available in the community in private practice.

~

So our medical profession has long had a code or principles of medical ethics, and now for some time they have even created a new form for medical and professional guidance: medical ethicists.

Let's remember what Dr. Makary had to say about the practice of medical ethics in his medical real world . . . in *Unaccountable*: *What Hospitals Won't Tell You and How Transparency Can Revolutionize Health Care.*

> Years after completing my medical training, I encountered one of my favorite public health professors, Harvard surgeon Dr. Lucian Leape, at a national surgeons' conference. He opened the gathering's keynote speech by looking out over the audience of thousands and asking the doctors to "raise your hand if you know of physician you work with who should not be practicing because he or she is dangerous." Every hand went up.
>
> Incredulous at this response, I took to asking the same question whenever I spoke at conferences. And I always got the same response. Every doctor knows about this problem—but few talk about it. Every day, people are injured or killed by a medical mistake that might have been prevented with a modicum of adherence to standardize guidelines. The silence about the problem has paralyzed efforts to address it—until now.

~

Dr. Lundberg recognized another highly credentialed physician with this comment: "Dr. Christine Cassel, another physician with a deep commitment to medical ethics, elaborated by listing ten characteristics of a learned professional, and we published them in *JAMA*: Self-governance individually and as a group."

Dr. Cassel will be the third NQF president and CEO (July 2013), replacing the recently retired Janet Corrigan, PhD.

Medical Ethics/Medical Peer Review

If medical ethics is self-governance individually and as a group, where does medical peer review come into play within the medical profession? Medical peer review is where one *must begin* when searching for medical ethics, because a medical profession without a functional system of medical peer review is a non-profession. (Revisit Dr. Makary's book, *Unaccountable*.)

I have always believed that medical peer review should be the center-pole for every consideration regarding medical ethics. Yet search the Centers for Medical Ethics, and now the schools training medical ethicists for evidence of medical peer review consideration. AMA Principles of Medical Ethics recognizes the need, but no one can find evidence of its reality within our current medical profession.

I have indicated in all three of my books that I can supply our medical profession with a system of medical peer review fair to both doctor and patient. So far, there has been no response from within our medical profession for more detailed information regarding my offer. Perhaps Doctors DeAngelis and Cassel and I could collaborate on a further study regarding the ethical obligation and responsibility of a true profession.

I can also provide a very simple test to demonstrate that meaningful medical peer review does not exist in any hospital medical staff in America. Problem: that test could only be conducted if I was provided with sufficient delegated authority to ask questions and demand definitive answers from the proper authorities in each hospital. That test would also NOT require piercing the curtain of secrecy under the current, counter-productive HCQIA-86 decree that allow all 50 state legislatures make medical peer review secret.

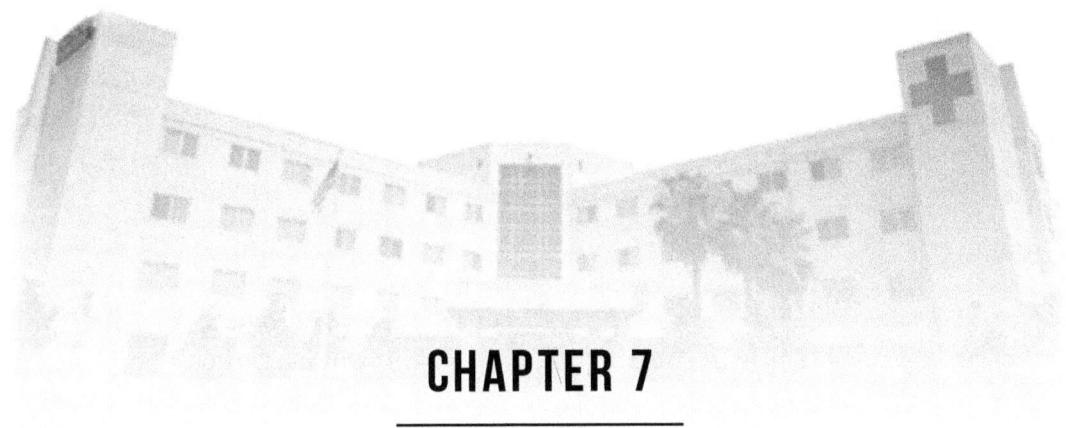

CHAPTER 7

TIMELINE CHECKLIST

Timelines provide a quick, broad perspective of the historical context of concerted effort throughout a protracted process involving the same, or similar issues. The benefits of checklists have been proven in the military and in healthcare. A timeline checklist of the broad spectrum of efforts to make healthcare safer provides an interesting perspective.

A starting point in 1986 illustrates widely divergent examples.

1986

Harvard Medical School Department of Anesthesia set fundamental "Minimal Standards for Patient Monitoring" that could be achievable even in the smallest rural community hospital. Their simple seven lines in the sand provided greatly improved patient safety within one year.

Brennan, Leape, and others at Harvard School of Public Heath began their four-year research study in New York hospitals, which eventually led to the accepted estimate of 98,000 needless hospital deaths annually used as the baseline for the IOM's report: *To Err Is Human*.

1988

Institute of Healthcare Improvements (IHI) (newly founded by Dr. Don Berwick and a group of visionaries committed to redesigning healthcare into a system without errors, waste, delay, and unsustainable costs) held their first annual meeting.

The AMA/Specialty Society Medical Liability Project was publicly announced for the creation of special medical malpractice courts. (The project died in mid-1990s.)

The *Wall Street Journal* reported that The Joint Commission hospital review service was discontinued by New York State after the state was forced to close a hospital shortly after it was accredited by The Joint Commission.

1990

Harvard School of Public Health experts (Brennan, Leape, and others) after four years of research, estimated that the number of needless deaths in our nation's hospitals was estimated to be 98,000 annually.

1995

"Bill" died in a North Carolina hospital under questionable circumstances (but his death would not go unnoticed).

1997

IOM patient safety studies began (which led to, *To Err Is Human* and *Crossing the Quality Chasm*).

AMA created National Patient Safety Foundation (after abandoning their failed efforts to create special medical malpractice courts).

AMA House of Delegates pass the first of four parliamentary votes that led to the creation of the Litigation Center.

Bill's parents settled malpractice claims against the hospital and 1st surgeon, and chose not to pursue further litigation against 2nd surgeon.

1998

National Quality Forum (NQF) was established by Congress to promote the quality, appropriateness, and effectiveness of healthcare.

1999

IOM first presented the report "To Err is Human," noting that, "Given current knowledge about the magnitude of the problem, the committee believes it would be irresponsible to expect anything less than a 50 percent reduction in errors over five years."

"The External Review of Hospital Quality, Holding the Reviewers Accountable, a five-part report, was issued by the Department of Health and Human Services, Office of Inspector General, Office of Evaluation and Inspection (Boston Regional Office) to assess how the Healthcare Financing Administration holds The Joint Commission and state agencies accountable for the external review of hospital quality. [NOTE: This five-part review report (with comments from The Joint Commission, Association of Health Facility Survey Agencies, American Osteopathic Association, American Association of Retired Persons, Service Employees International Union, National health Law Program, and Public Citizen's Health Research Group) was a *monumental* disgrace.]

2000

The book, *To Err Is Human,* was published, saying, "Given current knowledge about the magnitude of the problem, the committee believe it would be irresponsible to expect anything less than a 50 percent reduction in errors over five years."

AMA-State Medical Societies began creation of the Litigation Center

2001

Dr. Kenneth Kizer, NQF first president and CEO, introduced the term, *never events*, in reference to particularly shocking medical errors (such as wrong-site surgery) that should *never* occur.

2002

AMA-North Carolina Medical Association was joined by North Carolina Medical Board of Examiners to revoke NC medical license of Bill's medical malpractice expert witness from the 1997 legal proceedings.

AMA President-Elect Donald Palmisano, MD, said in his *A Primer of Malpractice Law*, "To determine the standard of care, to determine the height of the 'low hurdles' in the race of patient care, the law requires a MINIMALLY acceptable level of care; thus my analogy to the 'low hurdle.'"

2003

AMA President Donald J. Palmisano, MD, JD, said on a CME video, "Doctors, under the law, if you're treating a patient and you fall below a standard of care set by the law, and those standards are determined by experts, and that directly causes damage to the patient, that's medical malpractice." On *NewsHour* (PBS) he said, "We do know that the liability system does not measure negligence."

AMA brochure, "Will Your Doctor Be There?" noted: "The primary cause of America's medical liability crisis is overzealous personal injury attorneys who put their pocketbooks before patients."

2004

Dr. Elizabeth McGlynn reported for the Rand Corporation that "Americans get substandard care for their aliments about half the time. Only a fundamental redesign of the health system will improve the situation."

The last of a series of six books, *Crossing the Quality of Chasm,* was published by IOM with 53 Recommendations.

2007

The National Patient Safety Foundation creates the Lucian Leape Institute to serve as a strategic think tank on matters related to patient safety.

2008

NQF reports that patient safety is *improving only 1 percent each year.*

According to AHRQ Director Dr. Carolyn Clancy, "Overall, the review of forty core quality measures found a 3.1 percent increase in the quality of care—the same rate of improvement as the previous two years."

2009

Lucian Leape, MD, and Janet Corrigan, PhD, MBA, presented "Reflection on the Past 10 Years: Why Have We Not Gotten Further?" to a limited non-public audience.

The *New York Times* published "10 Steps to Better Healthcare" by four physicians: Atul Gawande, Donald Berwick, Elliott Fisher, and Mark McClellan, saying, "But all medicine is local. And until a community confronts what goes on in its own population—to the point of actually seeking the data and engaging those who can solve the problem—nothing will change."

New England Journal of Medicine published "Balancing 'No Blame' with Accountability in Patient Safety" by Robert M. Wachter, MD, and Peter J. Pronovost, MD, PhD, on the subject of hand hygiene.

2010

Dr. Spence Taylor, chairman of General Surgery, Greenville Hospital System, and operations director of the new USC School of Medicine/ Greenville Development Team, said, "Even if you cured cancer, you couldn't get it to the people, because the medical system is broken."

This conversation occurred:

IW:	"How do you get your system of systems errors to all of the hospitals in the nation?"
	Dr. Wachter: "That's a problem."
IW:	"I can solve that problem."
Dr.	Wachter: [Silence]

Chosen as a pilot for national effort to improve surgical safety with efforts expected to reduce patient deaths by hundreds each year, South Carolina partnered with renowned surgeon, Dr. Atul Gawande, in introducing a Surgical Safety Checklist in every operating room in the state.

Patient-Centered Outcomes Research Institute (PCORI) was created by Congress.

IOM "Roundtable on Value and Science-driven Healthcare" convened stakeholders from across the healthcare field in a series of four two- day meetings titled: "The Healthcare Imperative: Lowering Costs and Improving Outcomes 2010." The Workshop Series Summary (over 600 pages) listed four sections, containing twenty-two segments and over seventy presentations, providing a glimpse into the enormous size and diversity of the QHC army of experts.

2011

Governor Haley and the South Carolina Legislature rejected my offer to provide them with a detailed report of every component of their current healthcare delivery system. The governor said she didn't have "the authority" to do so.

2012

Unaccountable: What Hospitals Won't Tell You and How Transparency Can Revolutionize Healthcare by Marty Makary, MD, was published.

A National Transportation Safety Board for Healthcare—Learning From Innovation by Charles R. Denham, MD, Chesley B. Sullenberger, III, MS, Dennis W. Quaid, and John J. Nance, JD, was published.

Captain Chesley B. "Sully" Sullenberger began pointing out "There are 200,000 preventable deaths each year in the US healthcare system ... like having twenty Boeing 747 airliners going down each week" in numerous media sources and healthcare related articles.

Physician Jonathan R. Welch's article, "As She Lay Dying: How I Fought To Stop Medical Errors from Killing My Mom," appeared in *Health Affairs*.

IHI held its 24th Annual Meeting in Orlando, Florida.

2013

Dr. Robert Wachter posted on his blog this article, "Is the Patient Safety Movement in Danger of Flickering Out?"

Dr. Wachter asked his question, and was unable to answer it, just as he was unable to answer my question to him: "How do you get your system of systems-errors to every hospital in the nation?" He was silent then, and remains silent regarding that most important question—even as people continue to needlessly die in hospitals and surgery centers throughout the country.

Dr. Wachter should have asked, "Is there any possible way for the current quality of healthcare efforts to ever become successful (regardless of the standards and measures used) if we have no means to make those efforts become reality *throughout* our nation's healthcare delivery system?

There is overwhelming evidence to support a conclusion of *NO!*

If that conclusion proves correct, the needless hospital death national tragedy will continue unabated. Perhaps the greatest tragedy is the apparent fact that, as citizens and within the highest levels of government, we remain passively accepting of this massive and needless loss of lives.

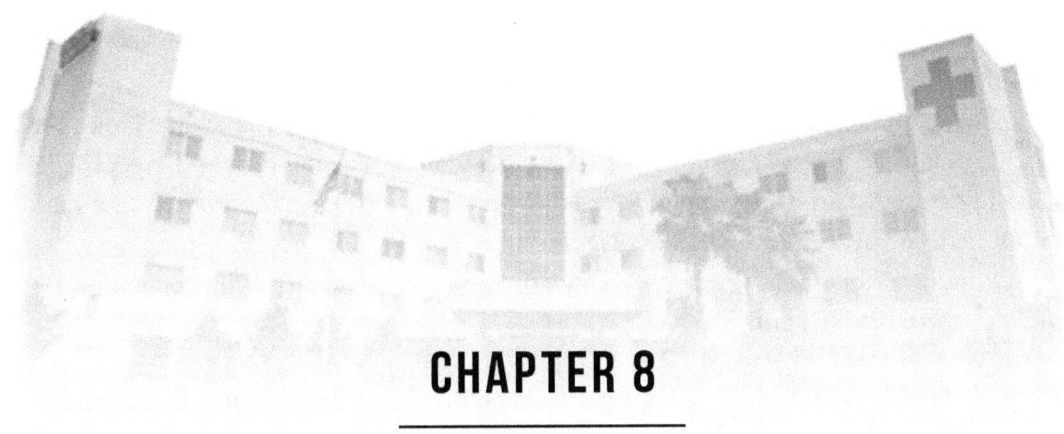

CHAPTER 8

THE SOLUTION

> All truth passes through three stages;
> First, it is ridiculed Second, it is violently opposed
> Finally, it is accepted as being self-evident.
> ~ Arthur Schopenhauer

Find the Black Box is predicated on the acceptance of two contrarian conclusions: Quality of healthcare experts have been unsuccessful in their efforts thus far due to their inability to recognize that each state is responsible for the creation and maintenance of an effective healthcare delivery system; and every state governor and legislature must recognize that the nation's healthcare delivery system can never function effectively while lacking an organizational structure, with clearly defined points of authority, delegated authority, and the resultant means for meaningful accountability.

Therefore, the solution necessary to vastly improve the entire healthcare delivery system requires that future efforts to improve the quality of healthcare in America be directed toward creating a state-based healthcare delivery system.

How to Begin the Solution Process

This is the detailed Proposal for Healthcare Change that would work in South Carolina, offered to Governor Haley.

Phase I: Governor Haley will hire a healthcare fact-finding consultant and authorize that consultant to meet with each identified agency, association, and organization currently acting as a component of South Carolina's current healthcare system, requesting full cooperation with the consultant from each participant.

The purpose of the healthcare fact-finding consultant is to describe in detail the organizational structure and function of the state's existing healthcare system. A role model for this task is the *Flexner Report* (1910), wherein Abraham Flexner reviewed every medical school in America and Canada, and his report resulted in the creation of the foundation for modern medical education in the US and later throughout Western Europe.

Duration of Phase I: Ninety (90) days would be sufficient with full cooperation from individual healthcare components.

Phase II: Governor Haley will assess the report and invite members of the various healthcare organizations subject to the Phase I study, and interested members of the public (and to be as open as possible to all interested parties), to summarize an overview of the status of healthcare in South Carolina and to consider the need for future change.

Duration of Phase II should be limited to ninety (90) days.

Phase III: Governor Haley will propose the creation of a "Big Tent" endeavor to begin the process of meaningful healthcare change in South Carolina, giving consideration to every source capable of contributing to that effort. The role model for this task is JFK's challenge to send men to walk on the moon and return them safely.

SC Healthcare System Components/Participants

> Arnold School of Public Health Carolina Center for Medical Excellence DHEC
> DHHS
> DNV—Healthcare
> Health Sciences for SC (HSSC) Medical Examining Board
> Medical School of SC Moore School of Business QIO (2)
> Quality Improvement Council
> SC Governor's Quality Award/Baldrige SC Hospital Association
> SC Medical Associations SC Medical School
> The Joint Commission

Healthcare Fact-finding Committee

Each organization must be reassured that the Healthcare Fact-finding Committee's intent is purely positive, and that great detail is required in order to provide the governor with a complete understanding of the state's current healthcare system. In order to create a complete picture of the organizational structure and method of functioning of the state's current healthcare system, individual represented components will describe:

- How they function individually.
- How they function within the healthcare system as a whole.

- What they can do to make healthcare safer.
- What they would like to be able to do to make healthcare safer.
- What they are unable to do to make healthcare safer.
- Their vision of a far more functional and efficient state healthcare system.
- Their willingness to fully cooperate in future efforts to make healthcare in South Carolina safer and more efficient.

Proposed Pre-meeting Agenda (sent prior to each meeting)

Clarify that due to the broad, fact-finding obligation of this committee, some of the requests for information may exceed the individual organization's purview. No undue pressure shall be implied or intended. The Committee's goal in seeking, in as much detail as possible, what each healthcare organization can and cannot do is intended to help us fully describe and understand the current organizational structure and functioning methods of each component and its relationship to the overall healthcare system. The Committee's responsibility to each organization is to affirm the positive nature of this fact-finding endeavor and eliminate any concern about negative intention.

Governor Haley must receive full cooperation of every component of the state's current healthcare system in order to consider future efforts for beneficial healthcare change. The future impact stemming from this fact-finding process will culminate in remodeling efforts for meaningful healthcare change. Governor Haley will urge full cooperation in this effort from all participants.

Start with understanding these fundamentals of healthcare: All medical care is local, and the states license most doctors to practice their profession. Therefore, states are individually responsible to their citizens for the regulation and control of the private practice of medicine, hospital medical staffs, and surgery centers. (No state can currently demonstrate an effective regulatory mechanism to fulfill that responsibility.)

Support Materials for Meaningful Healthcare Change

The Flexner Report is important because Abraham Flexner laid the foundation for modern medical education: First, one must know where we are now and how we got here prior to attempting to make meaningful change in large systems.

The US Department of Defense is important because it possesses an organizational structure with clearly defined points of authority, responsibility, and accountability. The absence of meaningful accountability is the root cause of the inability to improve the quality of healthcare.

The Moon Landing is important because numerous segments of varying expertise united under one "big tent" to overcome all of the obstacles impeding ultimate success. No one who expressed the ability to recognize the "impossible" were allowed admittance.

Welfare Change in Wisconsin is important because Governor Thompson and the state's Welfare Division demonstrated that, in spite of predictions of bodies in the streets due to death by starvation, the massive welfare system could successfully endure radical change.

MADD is important because they proved that a group of concerned citizens, acting in unison, could force the South Carolina Legislature to reconfigure a regulatory mechanism and achieve positive results.

Quality of Healthcare Realities in SC to consider:

- "Even if you cured cancer you couldn't get it to the people because the medical system is broken." ~ Dr. Spence Taylor, GHS chairman of the Department of Surgery. (April 2010)
- The South Carolina Hospital Association (SCHA) is embarking on a patient safety program that can potentially save hundreds of patient lives each year and reduce the number of major surgical complications up to 30 percent. SCHA serves 80 percent of the state's hospitals—and none of the surgery centers.
- The first large study in a decade to analyze harm from medical care and to track it over time, conducted from 2002 to 2007 in ten North Carolina hospitals, found that harm to patients was common and that the number of incidents did not decrease over time. Efforts to make hospitals safer for patients are falling short.
- The healthcare quality chasm is real, it is growing, it is costly; and there is *no* evidence that current efforts to reverse that deadly trend are having any positive effect. We must confront this issue forcibly.

Fundamental Flaws in this Offer to Governor Haley

State governors lack the authority to "appoint" fact-finding committees, and that inability is apparently shared by state legislatures. State governors and legislatures can jointly hire a consulting firm to conduct such a study, but they must first collectively recognize the need and create the will to do so.

State governors and legislatures should be forced to find hard evidence that would allow them to deny (in the face of the facts that all medical care is local, and that states license doctors) that "they" are not responsible for their state's healthcare delivery system. The simple fact is: every state has a healthcare delivery system, and no governor or state legislator can find even one person in their state with the ability to describe in detail that state's healthcare delivery system, name each component, describe how each component functions, and describe how or whether two or more of those components functions in a "systematic manner."

Patient safety and questionable patient care accountability are the key targets for any meaningful improvement in the quality of healthcare. Those joined-at-the-hip goals can never be attained unless medical peer review replaces medical malpractice litigation as the system of choice for the review of questionable patient care.

The following is a transcript of a fifteen-minute audio CD I produced in 2007:

The Two Missing Links of Medical Malpractice

Medical malpractice—is it?—or isn't it? How can we know? Let me open with a poorly recognized fact which hopefully will crystallize the immense depth of this problem. I offer three unfortunate events that could occur in any community in our nation tomorrow. However, these events did occur—at different times—in my community.

- A construction worker is accidentally killed at the worksite. OSHA investigators are on the scene within hours.
- A single-engine airplane crashes on takeoff. Both occupants walk away with only slight injuries. FAA investigators are at the site within hours.
- A twenty-seven-year-old slender, healthy wife and mother enters the hospital operating room for minor knee surgery under local anesthesia. She is injected once in the upper thigh area in front and once in the buttocks. Within minutes, she suffers a catastrophic systems collapse and within a few additional minutes she is clinically dead!

No investigators from any regulatory body ever appeared at the site of that tragedy. The widowed husband and father was forced to sue the doctors in order to find out *what* happened. On the third anniversary of the woman's death, a lay-jury returned a verdict of no negligence! The doctors had won another court case.

Two significant factors must be gained from that tragic, but true, story:

First, hospitals are the only places in America where an accidental death can occur and receive no regulatory, in-depth investigation by a state source of authority. How frightening! And *second,* the practice of medicine is one of the least regulated economic activities in America. Doctors are the best judges of other doctors, but doctors do not know *how* to judge other doctors.

Malpractice happens! Doctors are only human, and all humans make mistakes; even the best doctors make mistakes. The big problem is not that medical malpractice happens—it's inevitable. The big problem is our medical profession's failure to fairly judge questionable patient care within their profession. The issue should not be "medical malpractice." Rather, the issue is "questionable patient care"—and how doctors can fairly judge questionable patient care.

History plays an important part in understanding medical malpractice. Throughout American history, the practice of medicine has been a poorly regulated activity. Medical malpractice first became a recognized crisis in the mid-1800s, and almost all in-depth review of questionable patient care since that time has occurred before a judge and lay (non-medical) jury. The obvious root cause of that malpractice crisis remains puzzlingly obscure.

Doctors are by far the best judges of other doctors, and therefore it makes sense that they should be the best judges of questionable patient care. But, doctors have never created a system whereby they can fairly judge other doctors regarding questionable patient care.

Sometimes the obvious escapes notice! Our medical profession has one gigantic failure lurking in our otherwise marvelous history of modern medicine: They have never created a system whereby doctors can fairly judge the questionable patient care of another doctor, without attorneys, courts, and juries. This failure is compounded by the fact that there is zero evidence that our profession has ever even made a determined effort to create such a system.

From a tonsillectomy to a heart transplant, all medical treatments have several common, basic elements. Three of those basic elements are science, art, and standard of care.

All doctors are taught the *science* of medicine in medical school. All doctors provide the *art* of medicine. More precisely, each doctor provides his or her personal art of medicine to each patient they treat. Each patient is a fresh canvas demonstrating that doctor's art of medicine.

The perfect analogy for the practice of medicine is a pilot flying a single-engine airplane. Each student pilot is taught the science of flying an airplane. Each pilot, student or graduate pilot, provides their personal art of flying an airplane each time they take off and hopefully land safely. The exact same combination of science and art occurs every time a doctor treats a patient.

This basic understanding exposes a major component of the medical malpractice dilemma, and that is, all medical treatment is a combination of science and art; but the medical profession, as of today, has never been able to identify and define, and more importantly judge, the art of medicine involving the simplest form of patient care.

That fact, the medical profession's inability to identify, define, and judge one of the two basic characteristics of every form of medical care, is the first missing link in the medical malpractice crisis.

Standard of Care is the second missing link in the malpractice crisis. Just as every form of medical care is a combination of science and art, every form of medical care has a standard of care automatically attached to it. A doctor cannot treat a patient, in any manner, without there being a standard of care associated with that treatment.

The question that is fair to ask: "Doctor, when you treated this patient, what was your standard of care for that treatment?"

"What was the standard of care?" is a critical question, which must be answered in every review of questionable patient care.

Now that I have identified the two missing links in the medical malpractice crisis (finding the art of medicine and what is the standard of care), let's briefly review: As stated earlier, medical malpractice happens, but not all questionable patient care is medical malpractice. So, how can we judge what questionable patient care is medical malpractice and what questionable patient care is not medical malpractice?

Currently, there are three different systems used for the review of questionable patient care:

State medical examining boards. Data from the Federation of State Medical Boards show that system is rarely used for the review of individual cases of questionable patient care. The potential for such use does exist, but in name only!

Medical peer review. Doctors review the patient care of other doctors. Peer-review can occur at several levels of organized medicine, but the most effective system of medical peer review should occur at the hospital medical staff level. Does medical peer review occur in hospital medical staffs? Probably not! Why? Because Congress and the state legislatures made medical peer review totally secret! Medical peer review is more secret than almost anything non-military. Yes, medical peer review does exist. But like fog, there is no discernible substance and no identifiable benefit to society. Medical peer review and the state medical board's review of questionable patient care both exist essentially in name only!

Medical malpractice litigation (Sue or forget it.). This is at the center of all public debate regarding questionable patient care. Sadly, if medical peer review functioned properly, it would result in the need for far less medical malpractice litigation.

All three systems demand that the state board reviewers, medical peer review committee, and/or the civil court judge or jury create the medical standard of care they are to judge by.

The central point of this discussion: the AMA definition of medical malpractice is treatment *beneath the standard of care set by the law!* Where does that leave society? There can be no medical treatment given by a doctor to a patient without that treatment having a medical standard of care. Yet the AMA defines medical malpractice as *treatment beneath a standard of care set by the law.* Doctors do not know how to judge other doctors! Yet there is NO medical malpractice without medical expert witness testimony. The root cause of the medical malpractice problem is created by that professional dilemma. Until and unless doctors create a system whereby they can fairly judge other doctors regarding questionable patient care, the medical malpractice crisis will continue to exist and continue to grow.

However, such a system whereby doctors *can* fairly judge other doctors without attorneys, courts, and juries is far more attainable than imagined. I know this, because I can provide such a system.

Just as water requires two hydrogen and one oxygen molecules, all medical treatment requires the science and the art of medicine to result in a standard of care. A doctor's standard of care for every form of treatment he or she provides can only be found by reviewing the three elements in detail.

How?

The science of every form of medical treatment can be written to mimic the format of a single-engine airplane checklist. No person should willingly submit to surgery performed by a doctor who is unable/unwilling to document the scientific elements of their personal standard of care for the planned surgical procedure.

Doctors are never required to document the scientific elements of the standard of care they have been taught and are using in the daily performance of their profession. Yet the scientific elements of every medical standard of care, when combined, create the center pole of any system of review of questionable patient care. You can't have one, medical treatment—without the other, a standard of care.

Doctors created the medical malpractice litigation crisis by their failure to create a system whereby doctors (the best judges) could judge other doctors without attorneys, courts, and juries. That is why society has always been left with "Sue or forget it!" Attorneys filled the vacuum the doctors created by their own failure!

The AMA states that, "The primary cause of America's medical liability crisis is overzealous personal injury attorneys who put their pocketbooks before patients." Now ask yourself, if a person has surgery and, in time, reasonable questions arise, that happens, right? Then how, when, and where did an attorney create the problem? The AMA has no answer for that question.

Decades ago, doctors failed to recognize the fatal flaw of not creating a system of medical peer review which could complement the marvelous scientific achievements of their profession. Leaving society with "Sue or forget it," physicians drove a stake into the heart of their own profession. Only a system of medical peer review, fair to both doctor and patient, can ever right that wrong.

Our medical profession must redefine the definition of medical malpractice to treatment beneath a standard of care set by doctors (not the law).

Medical peer review, or more precisely, functional and meaningful medical peer review, must supply the *foundation* for an effective and efficient state healthcare delivery system. Anyone who believes they can create *practice standards* and *evidence-based medicine* formulated by far-removed quality of healthcare experts that are supposed to "trickle down" and throughout the entire system of hospitals and surgery centers in fly-over America (while "Sue or forget it" remains the system of choice for the review of questionable patient care) are delusional. A system for meaningful medical peer review forms the foundation that THE SOLUTION to our healthcare delivery system must rest upon.

My System for Meaningful Hospital Medical Staff Medical Peer Review

The Individual Responsibility Peer Review System (IRPR) amounts to four letters and a few easy steps, but how can doctors be convinced or forced into taking them?

An IRPR system says to every individual doctor, "Doctor, you take care of the person you see in the mirror each morning, and the IRPR system will take care of the medical malpractice problem."

Questionable patient care is a natural by-product of the practice of medicine. Why? Because the practice of medicine is one human treating another human using advanced scientific technologies. *All humans make human mistakes.*

No system of questionable patient care review will eliminate that part of the human equation. So, the next best alternative is to create a system of review that is as fundamentally sound as humanly possible, and fair to both doctor and patient. Any system that does not balance the scales of fair review equally, between both doctor and patient, will lack credibility and professional integrity. An IRPR system, properly organized and justly administered, can provide both of those absolute necessities.

The "ON" Button: Probably every hospital medical staff in America would claim they have either:

- standing departmental peer review committees, and/or
- a standing hospital medical staff peer review committee, and/or
- a hospital medical staff peer review system.

With medical peer review legislatively made secret, no details of past or present medical staff peer review functions can be discussed. You would think that federal and state legislatures might begin to wonder exactly what benefits to society are obtained by that collective agreement to secrecy.

Do systems of hospital medical staff peer review exist? *Yes.*

Do they function on a regular basis and in a systematic manner?

NO!

Why? This basic professional obligation to society lacks an "ON" button. Pressing it is equal to initiating the review process. Any hospital medical staff claiming to have an existing medical staff peer review system should be able to describe, in detail, the person or persons who are allowed to initiate activity within that system.

I initiated medical staff peer review activity in the three private hospitals in Madison, Wisconsin, and the University of Wisconsin Hospital and Clinics where I practiced. While each hospital medical staff responded differently, they were all less than professional. During my first experience in requesting medical peer review, as the second surgeon for that patient's original treatment (which was exceedingly negligent), I was asked by that hospital's medical director, "Are you a troublemaker?"

It's far too easy to rapidly pass over the question that goes right to the heart of the matter, and that everyone involved in seeking higher quality healthcare should be required to answer. Was I, or any other well-intended practitioner, acting as a troublemaker? America's healthcare system has been for far too long in this quality chasm quandary precisely because too few people have been asking the "hard questions."

A medical peer review system cannot be said to truly exist where no one can identify who is eligible to hit that system's "on" button, or even to hit that button knowing that there will be a price to pay. I paid that price.

Organized medicine cannot identify a proven medical peer review track record anywhere in America because they will not tolerate practitioners who might initiate that system, and because doctors don't know how to judge other doctors if such a system were to be initiated. Hospital administrations and medical staff leaders go into spasms the rare times they are forced, and that is the only way it can occur—to respond to such a request.

Activators of the IRPR System:

The "on" button must be accessible to individuals medically qualified or legally justified to do so.

Legally justified includes patient, spouse, immediate family member, or legal guardian.

Medically qualified: Hospital medical staff members and hospital employees having direct patient care responsibilities such as OR, ICU, and ER nurses, etc.

Only a hospital medical staff dedicated to the ethical foundation of their profession and to the community they have chosen to serve can create, establish, and fairly administer an IRPR system.

America has an estimated 5,000 or more hospitals; and those hospitals and their medical staffs are like 5,000 or more different people. They all differ in size, makeup, personalities, etc. The IRPR system can be modified into equally differing sizes and shapes to fit the needs of each hospital medical staff. But fundamental elements of the system must remain the same in every IRPR system of questionable patient care review.

After an IRPR system is firmly established and the medical staff members see a system that can fairly judge questionable patient care, the treating doctors may even be willing, at times, to activate the system for review of their own patient care. Malpractice litigation denies a doctor the review of their personal track record of patient care, which would be the best means of identifying good doctors who will occasionally make common, human mistakes. The competent physician's best friend can be found in a properly functioning IRPR system of peer review. The poorly qualified physician's worst nightmare can be found in that exact same system.

Medical Staff Peer Review Coordinator: An IRPR system, once activated, must have a gatekeeper. Staffing this position will vary by hospital size and medical staff makeup. Medical staff designation of such a person may range from the chief of Staff or medical director at larger hospitals to possibly even a highly qualified nurse at smaller hospitals.

The key issue is that the peer review coordinator has unquestionable authority and the full support of the hospital administration and medical staff in order to fulfill the obligations of that position. Resistance to proper response to requests from the peer review coordinator by any medical staff member cannot, and must not, be tolerated.

A properly functioning IRPR system can never be created and utilized unless it is clearly understood that every physician on the medical staff, from the chief of Staff down to the newest member, may be subject to IRPR review if they are actively treating patients at that hospital. Any deviation from that understanding will render an IRPR system a sham.

Medical Staff Member Subject to Peer Review: After the Peer Review coordinator has responded to system's activation and made sufficient inquiry and medical record review to establish a need for full IRPR review, the medical staff member will be notified that such review will be rapidly undertaken.

IRPR review is a review of a practitioner's personal patient care track record; therefore, *at least* three patient care medical records will be included in the review process. Should red flags become evident during the initial review process, additional patient care records of similar types of treatment will be added to the review.

One of the most insidious forms of negligent patient care is the use of outdated, substandard methods of care. An IRPR system of peer review offers organized medicine an opportunity to raise the bar of patient care from the legally acceptable medical standard of care presently "set at the lowest possible hurdle" to a far more professional current and acceptable standard of care level. It is in the zone of medical practice located between those two differing standards of care that the unqualified and marginally qualified practitioners will be identified.

The medical staff member to be reviewed will supply the following for purposes of that review:

1. Documentation of personal training and experience necessary for that form of patient care (on an as-needed basis).
2. All outpatient medical records, photos, laboratory reports, x-rays, etc., associated with the treatment of the three similar cases being reviewed, with the understanding that additional cases will be reviewed if indicated.
3. Treatment-specific informed consent forms, i.e., a total-hip- replacement patient would be given a total-hip-replacement informed consent form prior to surgery.
4. A signed affidavit of cooperation. Every medical staff member of a hospital having an IRPR system of peer review will be required to have signed an affidavit offering full cooperation when the subject of IRPR review and full participation when requested to serve as a reviewer.
5. A detailed, itemized checklist of the scientific elements of that practitioner's personal standard of care for the specific form of medical care being reviewed.

The list of scientific elements for the treatment being reviewed allows doctors of different specialties to fairly peer review other doctors. For instance, a peer review committee made up of an internist, a general surgeon, and an urologist can fairly peer review an orthopedic surgeon. Any person who can master sufficient knowledge of neuroanatomy and biochemistry to graduate from medical school can follow the steps of a standard of care checklist and compare those to what actually occurred as noted in the patient's medical record.

Treatment-specific standard of care checklists and the multiple, personal track record patient care reviews are where organized medicine can begin to separate the qualified practitioners from the unqualified. Once a properly functioning IRPR system of peer review has been established long enough to demonstrate fair medical peer review is possible, the qualified practitioners should feel a great weight lifted from their mental shoulders. It is like saying, "Doctor, go and practice the kind of medicine you are personally capable of."

> ***Insight:*** Every practicing physician who has no single engine flight experience should go take at least two flying lessons. The purpose is to experience the difference between the science and the art of flying an airplane. Then they can translate that experience into a much deeper understanding of the difference between the science and art of medicine; then incorporate that new appreciation of the two indispensable characteristics of all medical care into their personal care of every future patient.
>
> The airplane checklist provides the scientific elements of flying a particular type of airplane from preflight, start engine and take off, to landing and engine off.

The medical standard of care must cease to be some nebulous, theoretical entity and become a clearly definable medical truth. Standard is defined as a rule used as a basis for judgment. The quality chasm has long existed because the medical standard of care has never fulfilled the promise of that definition.

Peer Review Committee: At least three medical staff members are necessary for this IRPR requirement. At first it may be viewed as a thankless job, but someone has to do it. Once firmly established, it will be an opportunity to establish the practice of medicine as a true profession in the eyes of that local community. The practice of medicine will take on a new meaning.

To establish an IRPR system initially, a hospital medical staff will probably be forced to form multiple three-member peer review teams created by lot drawn, or some other reasonable method. Those committees have an equal obligation to both doctor and patient.

Each peer review committee member will take one of the three initial patient care cases and a copy of the practitioner's standard of care checklist, and then do a step-by-step review of that patient's care. The best advice a Peer Review Committee member can receive is, "Let the chips fall where they may." Peer Review Committee members are neither practitioner's protectors nor patient's advocates. They represent *all of the above!*

Time is of the essence. Patient care review demands a prompt response from all parties involved. Peer Review Committee members who are less than diligent or biased toward doctors must be censored in the strongest manner. The professional integrity of that local medical community rests in their hands.

The three Peer Review Committee members will meet and jointly review each member's findings. Red flags will be noted for sufficient indication that additional patient care medical records should be added to the review process. It is imperative that the treatment-specific patient care track record of every medical staff member being reviewed be of a *current* and *acceptable* nature. Outmoded patient care techniques must be identified and eliminated for the benefit of the local community.

A joint meeting of the Peer Review Committee and the staff member being investigated will be held following sufficient review of multiple patient care records. A list of concerns and questionable patient care items will be presented to them as necessary. Favorable findings of quality patient care will also be noted.

The IRPR system allows a hospital medical staff to differentiate between acceptable patient care with complications and negligent patient care (a major failing that medical malpractice litigation can never satisfy). No other system of questionable patient care review judges a practitioner's art of medicine and allows a doctor's patient care track record to demonstrate that doctor's quality of care. Here, too, is where the medical staff can discover those practitioners who may have added new patient care procedures to their personal scope of practice without proper credentialing or qualification.

The medical staff member being reviewed will be asked to review in detail any questionable items regarding:

- pre-treatment diagnosis and treatment planning;
- treatment-specific aspects of patient care including elements of surgeries or invasive procedures involved within that treatment;
- post-treatment aspects of patient care;
- need for consultations;*
- complications, actual and/or anticipated as highly possible;
- subject member's summation of all events that led to the IRPR review process;
- clarification of differences of opinion between subject member and the committee findings; and
- Peer Review Committee reports to the peer review coordinator.

*Consultations demand specific requirements:

- All consultations are requested from qualified sources who accept the consultation obligation.
- All requests for consultations are noted in the patient's medical record with documentation of need for the consultation and medical support sought.
- Acceptance by the consultant is noted in the patient's medical record.
- Detailed findings by the consultant are noted in the patient's medical record.

The Patient's Medical Record: There are two very important fundamentals of every patient's medical record that should be understood by those seeking to improve the quality of healthcare through the review of questionable patient care.

The combination of the patient and their medical record provides the "art" of an individual practitioner's art of medicine. Also, the patient medical record is one of the most abused aspects of the practice of medicine anywhere in America today. [It would take someone only minutes in any hospital medical record department to find numerous examples of negligent documentation of specific patient care. Furthermore, AMA, TJC, all state hospital associations, and particularly, all hospital medical record department staff, know that to be true; and that outrage has been passively accepted.]

The unwritten rule regarding patient's medical records is: If it's not written, it didn't occur. Negligent documentation is the first shortcoming found in many, if not most, patient medical records. Unadulterated arrogance in the form of illegible orders and progress notes scrawled across the page exude contempt and is common in medical records.

If you want to see the perfidy of healthcare in America, take a close look at numerous patient medical records shortly after a hospital has received a clean bill of health from The Joint Commission. They talk of having accountability when meaningful accountability is not evident. Hospitals advertise cardiovascular surgery, orthopedic surgery, OB-GYN surgery, and others "to a higher standard."

If they know the present treatment is to a "higher standard," then they must know the previous standard. Yet the AMA defines malpractice as treatment beneath a standard of care "set by the law." If one were ever allowed to closely review fifty patient medical records of any specialty claiming patient care to a higher standard, I believe those ads would disappear.

Accountability, standards, peer review, and other terms used to describe current medical care in America have no fundamental support in fact. The practice of medicine is among the least regulated economic activities in America, and organized medicine provides the least amount of factual accountability.

This brief description of an IRPR system of medical peer review may unintentionally mislead some into assuming it to be too simplistic for the task it is meant to accomplish. The deficiency lies in the form of presentation. The most comprehensive way to be introduced to the IRPR system would be by using a live audience of open-minded people seeking ways to improve the existing healthcare system.

The IRPR system of medical peer review can be expanded far beyond current imagination. Only a live audience presentation with audience participation can first demonstrate that system's full potential.

Medical malpractice litigation is and has been the primary system utilized by organized medicine for the review of questionable patient care. Doctors and patients deserve a far better system of patient care review. Civil court litigation is conducted under the restraints of "rules of evidence" and other legal hindrances to rational review. Frequently, obvious questions cannot be asked, or answers given, unless a legal foundation for that line of questions has been established. Civil court legal limitations can easily befuddle all listeners except the judge and attorneys present. It is nearly impossible to fairly judge the diverse essentials of questionable patient care through civil court litigation, yet lay jurors are asked to do just that.

There are no rules of evidence in an IRPR system of medical peer review. Doctors may talk freely, using professional terms. Straightforward questions should be asked, and straightforward answers should ensue.

Society must be protected from doctors who cannot or will not demonstrate the ability to rationally present what they did to a patient, how they did it, and why they did it as they did. Medical peer review is the only cure for the medical malpractice crisis; and no, attorneys are not the primary cause of that crisis, regardless of what the AMA says.

Consider this contrast in reasoning:

- Medical malpractice litigation is a system despised by doctors and patients.
- IRPR is a system that can restore doctors to being in charge of their profession, and would be the "good" doctors' best friend.

Benefits of the IRPR System

Doctor, how would you like to:

Set and control the quality of medicine practiced in your hospital?
Be judged by fellow practitioners using a system of peer review fair to both doctor and patient?
Identify, define, and judge the art of medicine?
Greatly reduce the need for the legal review of questionable patient care?
Practice your personal style of medicine knowing that, when necessary, your patient care will be judged upon your documented track record without attorneys, courts, or juries?
Restore confidence to the public you serve that they are cared for by members of a true profession that offers fair review of patient care within their profession?
Practice your profession without fear of unreasonable accusations?
Utilize standards of care set by the medical profession and not by the legal system?

Every time I have attempted to speak with doctors about the IRPR system of medical peer review, I am met with instant, strong, negative exceptions as to why such a system is "impossible." Doctors practicing medicine in the litigious climate *they created* cannot comprehend a system of doctors *fairly* judging other doctors. A live presentation would allow them to be "walked through the entire process" prior to their making a judgment regarding its feasibility.

I have told a few people that my dream is to one day have an opportunity to present an all day presentation on my vision of what I now call The Big Tent phase of meaningful healthcare delivery system change. Since that "presentation" is only in my head, I feel I need to say it would take me a full day to present. However, that presentation would begin with my walking through the IRPR system of medical peer review, followed by a controlled and courteous, but robust, Q&A.

People, and particularly doctors, need to understand that that IRPR system is NOT some form of medieval torture. A doctor's best friend is his or her personal patient care track record, and medical peer review is the only one of the three potential systems for questionable patient care review that allows doctors to use and benefit from their own track records.

But IRPR medical peer review is only the beginning, even though a most important beginning, of my vision of a complete reorganization of any state's healthcare delivery system. My complete plan goes far beyond anything anyone has yet imagined.

Doctors are the ones (and only ones) who "made the Faustian bargain many years ago" that "divorced the accountability for the bad results from the clinicians who are really best situated to fix the problems that gave rise to the unanticipated outcome, and it foisted it to a profession that is built for fighting. We got just what we asked for, an adversarial process." (Mr. Boothman, in his conversation with Dr. Wachter) Far too many doctors are disenchanted with their *chosen* field of endeavor, because doctors long ago chose the easy way out for them and left society with "Sue or forget it."

A well-established IRPR system of medical peer review in every state's hospital medical staff will enable (force) state medical boards to finally fulfill their original mandate and become the active participant and key component in the real regulation of the practice of medicine. Every patient care practitioner, regardless of profession, would be brought into a unified system of practitioner regulatory control. That process is far easier to establish than anyone has imagined, but it is all dependent upon first establishing the IRPR system of medical peer review in every hospital medical staff.

There is more—far more!

State healthcare delivery systems can rapidly become the greatest source of medical research. The complete absence of an organizational structure, with clearly defined points of authority, delegated authority, and the resultant meaningful accountability, has led to the greatest healthcare system the world has ever known becoming a third-rate, chaotic mess of needless hospital deaths.

Compare my offer of a series of steps toward a meaningful solution to the solutions offered in other books regarding the quality of healthcare. I can only hope that, due to the established insufficient track record by the current army of quality of healthcare experts ("1 percent each year" improvement), my offer will receive consideration.

All of us need to clearly understand that the subject is our, our children's, and our grandchildren's healthcare delivery system—and that system does not play favorites. That system will, sooner or later, reach out and grab everyone.

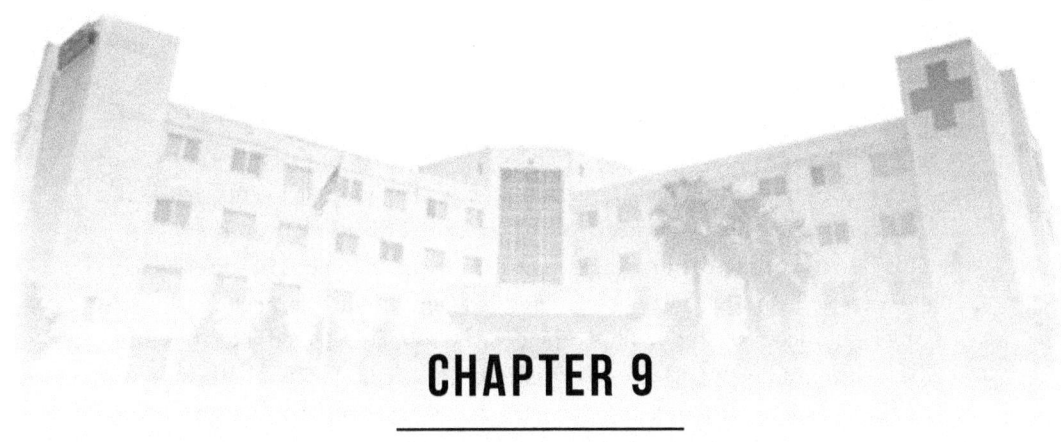

CHAPTER 9

CONCLUSION

I am an iconoclast and a contrarian, but thankfully, I am a positive contrarian. I have always sought ways to make our healthcare system "better" in my sphere of patient care. Unfortunately for my professional well being, I have spent too many years in the healing professions while they have continually lied to the public they sought to serve about their lack of professionalism. However, I don't expect people to take my word as proof of that indictment. Read what "they" say, or how "they" have been described by others.

Organized medicine was represented solely by the founding of the American Medical Association (AMA) in 1847, followed by the American College of Surgeons (ACS) in 1913, and the American College of Physicians (ACP) in 1915. Paul Starr best described the true measure of how doctors dominated healthcare in America throughout most of its history in *The Social Transformation of American Medicine*. I repeat from Chapter 5:

> Yet the replacement of a competitive orientation with a corporate consciousness required more than common interests. It required a transfer of power to the group, and this was what began to happen in medicine around 1900 with changes in its social structure. Physicians came increasingly to rely on each other's good will for their access to patients and facilities. Physicians also depended more on their colleagues for defense against malpractice suits, which were increasing in frequency.
>
> The courts, in working out the rules of liability for medical practice in the late nineteenth century, had set as the standard of care that of the local community where the physicians practiced. This limited possible expert testimony against physicians to their immediate colleagues. By adopting the "locality rule," the courts prepared the way for granting considerable power to the local medical society, for it became almost impossible for patients to get testimony against a physician who was a member. Medical societies began to make malpractice defense a direct service. Shortly after the turn of the century, doctors in New York, Chicago, and Cleveland organized common defense funds.

The Massachusetts Medical Society began handling malpractice suits in 1908. During the next ten years, it supported accused physicians in all but three of the ninety-four cases it received. Only twelve of these ninety-one cases went to trial, all save one resulting in a victory for the doctor. For its first twenty years, the defense fund of the medical society of the state of Washington won every case it fought. Because of their ability to protect their members, medical societies were able to get low insurance rates, while doctors who did not belong could scarcely get any insurance protection. This provided the sort of "selected incentive" that medical societies needed to help them attract members. Professional ostracism carried increasingly serious consequences: denial of hospital privileges, loss of referrals, loss of malpractice insurance, and in extreme cases, loss of a license to practice. The local medical fraternity became the arbiter of a doctor's position and fortune, and he could no longer choose to ignore it. By making the county societies the gatekeeper to membership in any higher professional group, the AMA had recognized and strengthened the position of the local fraternity, as well as bolstering its own organizational underpinnings.

Professor Starr described organized medicine during the same period that Abraham Flexner was publishing his *Report,* which began the process of creating the foundation for medical education throughout the civilized world. That process took several decades, but medical educators did a far better job of making medical education what it turned out to be than the leadership of practicing physicians ever attempted to do. Judge for yourself where is organized medicine now, a century later.

> "Those who cannot remember the past are
> condemned to repeat it."
>
> ~ George Santayana

We all know the healthcare system is broken, burdening our families, businesses, and national debt. It needs common-sense reform.

What will it take?

Our nation's healthcare delivery system does not need to be *re*organized. Our nation's healthcare delivery system has never been *organized* in the first place! Our nation's healthcare delivery system is a non-system, and our medical profession within that non-system does not behave as a true *profession*.

States license doctors and all medical care is local. Begin there.

States are responsible for our nation's healthcare delivery system. Unless governors and state legislators come to recognize *their inherent responsibility* to create and maintain an organized and functional healthcare delivery system for their respective citizens—and also create a system of meaningful accountability for our healthcare professionals, healthcare in America will remain in chaos.

Michelle M. Mello (an ardent supporter of Common Good and special malpractice courts) and Troyen A. Brennan (co-leader with Dr. Lucian Leape in the original research that estimated 98,000 needless hospital deaths annually in 1990) wrote about the role of medical liability reform in federal healthcare reform in 2009, saying, "The three reform approaches are not mutually exclusive and indeed could complement one another. All face a common legal hurdle: federalism. The fact that medical malpractice law has traditionally been controlled by the states complicates attempts to impose a federal structure on it. However, there are at least two ways Congress could surmount the federalism obstacle: declare its intent to completely preempt state regulation of the field—a drastic step—or simply condition states' receipt of federal health funds or "bonus payments" on their willingness to adopt changes to their tort systems.

Mello and Brennan have thrown down the gauntlet regarding who will dominate our nation's healthcare delivery system in the future. I find their challenge to be one of the most frightening proposals ever suggested regarding the regulation of patient care in America.

Governors, state legislators, and congressmen who support some semblance of state's rights must lead in this pending confrontation. If patient safety activists think the quality of healthcare is problematic now, just wait for the federal government to take complete control of the "regulation of the practice of medicine." That goes for the medical profession as well.

I have been (naively?) surprised that every nationally recognized patient safety activist (except one) has shunned my efforts to contribute to their cause. Apparently they have failed to recognize that I became a patient safety activist in 1979 when I forced every level of the St. Mary's Hospital Medical Staff and Administration, including the Sisterhood Headquarters in St. Louis, to confront the fact that two of their surgeons had provided grossly negligent care to a patient over a four-month period. I was well aware at the time that I was jeopardizing my professional career by doing so.

The basis for my original confrontation with the medical and hospital leadership in Madison, Wisconsin, followed by other, similar confrontations, and ultimately leading me to write three books on our healthcare delivery system, is really quite simple: I have always thought that patients have rights too. Unfortunately, such thinking (remember Semmelweis) is rarely, if ever, tolerated within any medical community in the nation.

Medical peer review is, and has always been, a non-entity in our nation's healthcare delivery system because the doctors in every medical community will not tolerate its existence. Organized medicine and hospital associations do NOT hold absolute control over any medical community that might choose to support a meaningful system of medical peer review. Patient safety activists plead for greater transparency and accountability in patient care, while at the same time, failing to recognize that medical peer review is the perfect vehicle by which to obtain those attributes.

New Jersey Law Revision Commission final report relating to medical peer review privilege in September 2005 said, "Medical peer review is a process whereby doctors evaluate the quality of work done by their colleagues, in order to determine compliance with accepted healthcare standards. This self-regulatory procedure provides quality assurance for the medical community by fostering standardization of appropriate medical procedures and by policing caregivers who could pose risks to patients. The rationale for the process is efficiency: working doctors are best situated to judge the competence of other working doctors because they regularly see each others' work and possess the relevant expertise to evaluate it."

"Peer review is one of the chief means of monitoring the quality of doctors' work"; the other two are state licensing board disciplinary action and tort law medical malpractice. Ideally, effective peer review should decrease the number of medical malpractice events and improve overall healthcare. Doctors, courts, and critics recognize the review process as an efficient means of professional self-regulation. Yet organized medicine convinced Congress in 1986, rapidly followed by every state legislature, to make medical peer review secret, "so that doctors could more freely talk about other doctors." We see how well that has gone.

My Offers for Meaningful Change First, *Find the Black Box*

States license doctors and each state's medical board is mandated to *regulate the practice of medicine* in their state. Therefore, somewhere, there should be a *regulatory mechanism* created for that purpose, but don't bet on it. That seemingly simple task would be like hitting each state's governor and legislature between the eyes with a two-by-four, and that is just what they need regarding their state's healthcare delivery system.

Every state has a regulatory mechanism for drunk driving that allows three different law enforcement agencies, city police, county sheriffs, and state patrol officers, to attempt to regulate driving under the influence. Because of MADD, we have clear evidence that state legislatures can, when forced to, find that regulatory mechanism and tinker with it. Problem is that no state governor or legislature will ever even look, unless forced to, for their state's practice of medicine regulatory mechanism—it's kept somewhere in a proverbial black box that should be in their medical examining board's office.

A chairman of the Department of General Surgery at a major medical center can say, "Even if we had a cure for cancer we couldn't get it to the people because the medical system is broken," and no decision maker or media watchdog even blinks an eye. Why? What he said was *not* news to them! Every person, in every state, knows their healthcare delivery system is broken, so why should they get excited just because some high-ranking doctor finally acknowledges the truth?

If governors and state legislatures responded each time someone with sufficient standing acknowledged the truth about serious matters, they (state decision makers) would be forced to confront those matters, and make hard decisions. (Decision makers cannot make too many hard decisions and continue to get reelected.)

What that high-ranking doctor didn't say was, "Why is the medical system broken?" Nor did he suggest that, perhaps, he and others should begin a process for "healing" that broken system. Isn't that what doctors are supposed to do, heal the sick and broken?

The fact remains, hospitals are the only place in America where an accidental death (regardless of the vast number) receives NO immediate review by a source of authority created by the state that licenses those doctors involved with that medical tragedy.

Next: My 3-Phase Process

1. Ask and answer: Where are we now and how did we get here?

Only a fool would attempt to change a huge system, particularly as important as healthcare, if they could not first benefit from having a detailed picture of that system, including every component, and the description of how they each function, both individually and collectively (a system). I can facilitate the creation of such a detailed picture of any state's healthcare delivery system within months (not years). But this requires being granted sufficient delegated authority and full-force backing by the combined authority of the governor and state legislature. No current component of any state healthcare delivery system is eager to provide a detailed picture of how they do their business now, and have been for years, simply because their component is broken, and they have been contributing to that combined failure.

The first state to engage in this 3-Phase Process would become the role model for every other state. Much of the total process would be just repetition for the second state. Then the ball would be rolling for meaningful healthcare change at the state level, where the quality of healthcare can rapidly gain its greatest benefit.

2. Assess the report and determine the next course of action.

Rest assured, the First Phase Report will provide an ugly picture, because every state's current healthcare delivery system is broken. We must manage our expectations. What the citizens of that state should expect is for their state's decision makers to accept reality and respond (act) in a responsible manner. Do something about it!

3. Allow me into the "Big Tent."

As with allowing men to walk on the moon and return safely, a wide variety of expertise will be necessary to finally create, for the first time, an organizational structure for their state's healthcare delivery system. I request the chance to present my vision for a state healthcare delivery system that, I guarantee, will go far beyond anything yet imagined.

Finally: Authority, Delegated Authority, and Meaningful Accountability

An effective and efficient healthcare delivery system is, and will continue to be, an impossible dream as long as civil litigation remains the system of choice for the review of questionable patient care. Organized medicine abdicated their professional responsibility to the legal profession over 150 years ago by only leaving the public with "Sue or forget it." Doctors must take back their professional responsibility. The only way they can do that is by adopting meaningful medical peer review.

My system of medical peer review is equally fair to both doctor and patient.

We all can agree that it is not easy judging the questionable patient care of another practitioner. Every time I testified against another surgeon, I reminded myself that I had a combined responsibility to:

- patient,
- surgeon,
- hospital medical staff,
- community,
- profession, and
- myself.

If enough doctors want to reclaim their profession from the legal profession, and only use "Sue or forget it" as a last resort in the review of questionable patient care, I can provide an equally fair system of medical peer review. The transition from that current, perverse system to one that captures the full essence of a true profession will not be easy, but well worth the effort. If doctors want to get back to enjoying the science and art of practicing medicine, they must be willing to make that necessary great effort.

Success in this endeavor will depend upon our ability to address difficult obstacles that are necessary to overcome for meaningful healthcare delivery system change:

1. Will state leaders continue to ignore their healthcare responsibility and, by such neglect, allow the federal government to continue to usurp and mismanage the affairs of our healthcare delivery system?
2. Can doctors reject "Sue or forget it" as the system of choice for the review of questionable patient care and recapture their profession and their professional obligation to the public through the use of meaningful medical peer review?

Ignaz Semmelweis offered one of the most fundamental necessities of quality healthcare: doctors must wash their hands and instruments. But his offer was rejected by those in the position to determine its acceptance.

Dr. Semmelweis did not *create* the *fact(s)* that doctors, by washing their hands and instruments could save lives. He *recognized* the positive results in patient safety that nuns, a few blocks away, were achieving, *tested* his theory, and *proved* the patient safety value achievable.

I did not *create* the facts regarding our healthcare delivery system; all medical care is local, states license doctors, and every state's medical examining board is over 100 years old. I did *recognize* those indisputable *facts*, and have devised a logical and doable process suitable to test the validity of those *facts*.

Medicine is a science, and one of the most inherent characteristics of true scientific endeavors has always been the absolute necessity to test new theories, particularly when current efforts are continuing to prove unproductive. Dr. Wachter's poignant plea, "Is the Patient Safety Movement in Danger of Flickering Our?" should support a sense of urgency throughout the entire quality of healthcare scope of effort the urgent need to consider alternative thinking. Semmelweis' disgraceful rejection by the medical leadership in two major European cities merely in an effort for those same medical leaders to "save face', rather than save lives should be a reminder to the quality of Healthcare Army of Experts.

And Sully Sullenberger's dramatic recognition of the current quality of healthcare throughout that entire "system" reflects the patient safety disparity Semmelweis encountered in child-birth in his day.

Addressing our abundance of needless hospital deaths is our current fundamental necessity for quality healthcare. Each state's responsibility to create and maintain an effective healthcare delivery system for their citizens is just as fundamental (based upon undeniable facts) as Semmelweis's offer more than 150 years ago. The stark resemblance between Semmelweis's time and today is due to the absence of a healthcare delivery system organizational structure with clearly defined points of authority, delegated authority, and all of the accountability benefits that can accompany such an absolute necessity. A truly scientific community would test this hypothesis.

Quality of healthcare, such as it is currently, deserves open consideration of all offers. With the utmost courtesy and respect, I offer the evidence and proposals in this book as a challenge to every governor and state legislature, the army of quality of healthcare experts, and all others who claim to have a stake in this most important issue.

Debate anyone?

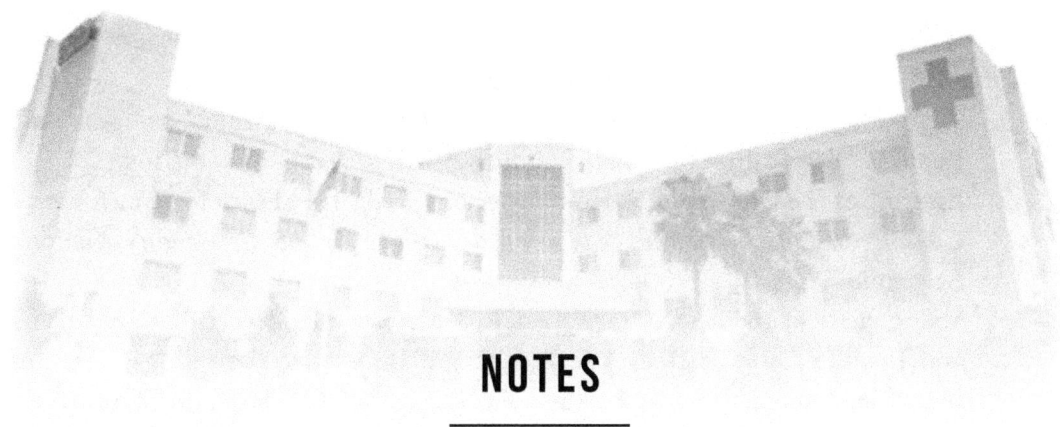

NOTES

Introduction
1. Brennan, Troyen A., Lucian L. Leape, Nan M. Laird, et al. "Incidence of adverse events and negligence in hospitalized patients: Results of the Harvard Medical Practice Study I." *New England Journal of Medicine*. 324:370–376, February 7, 1991. http://www. nejm.org/doi/full/10.1056/NEJM199102073240604.
2. Institute of Medicine (IOM), Linda T. Kohn, Janet M. Corrigan, and Molla S. Donaldson. *To Err Is Human: Building a Safer Health System*. Committee on Quality of Health Care in America, National Academies Press, 2000. *To Err Is Human: Building a Safer Health System*.
3. McGlynn, Elizabeth A., Steven M. Asch, John L Adams, et.al., "The Quality of Health Care Delivered to Adults in the United States, a two-year Rand Corporation study, *New England Journal of Medicine*, June 26, 2003, 348(26) 2635–2645.
4. Taylor, Dr. Spence. "Even if you cured cancer you couldn't get it to the people because the medical system is broken." *Greenville Journal*, April 2010.

Chapter 1: Who is Responsible?
1. Gawande, MD, Atul, Donald Berwick, Elliott Fisher, and Mark McClellan. "10 Steps to Better Healthcare" *New York Times* OP-ED Contributors, August 13, 2009.
2. Makary, MD, Marty. *Unaccountable: What Hospitals Won't Tell You and How Transparency Can Revolutionize Healthcare*. Bloomsbury Press, 2012.

Chapter 2: What's Missing?
1. Makary, MD, Marty. *Unaccountable: What Hospitals Won't Tell You and How Transparency Can Revolutionize Healthcare*. Bloomsbury Press, 2012.
2. Landro, Laura. "Hospital Horrors, Unaccountable," Marty Makary, MD, Bookshelf review, *Wall Street Journal*, October 4, 2012.

Chapter 3: Quality of Healthcare Army of Experts

1. *To Err Is Human: Building a Safer Health System.* http://www.iom.edu/Reports/1999/To-Err-is-Human-Building-A-Safer-Health- System.aspx.
2. Institute of Medicine (IOM). Committee on Quality of Health Care in America, *Crossing the Quality Chasm: A New Health System for the 21st Century.* National Academies Press, 2001-2004.
3. Young Pierre L. and LeighAnne Olsen, Roundtable on Evidence- Based Medicine, and Institute of Medicine. The Healthcare Imperative: Lowering Costs and Improving Outcomes. Workshop Series Washington DC: The National Academies Press. December 17, 2010.
4. http://www.ahrq.gov/
5. Wachter, MD, Robert M. *WebM&M* interview with NQF President Janet Corrigan, April 2010. http://www.webmm.ahrq. gov/
6. Wachter, MD, Robert M. "Is the Patient Safety Movement in Danger of Flickering Out?" *Wachter's World* blog. February 18, 2013
7. http://www.qualityforum.org/
8. Pronovost, P.M., M. Makary, et al., "Surgical never events in the United States." *Surgery Journal,* December 2012.
9. http://www.ihi.org/
10. http://www.pcori.org/.
11. http://www.scbch.org/
12. Sheridan, MIM, MBA, Susan S. and Martin J. Hatlie, JD. "We're Not Your Enemy: An Appeal from a Consumer to Re-imagine Tort Reform" *Patient Safety & Quality Healthcare Journal* July/ August 2007.
13. McMahan, Dr. Howard, "A day in the Life of a Country Doctor." *Parade,* March 3 2013.

Chapter 4: Quality of Healthcare Improvement Experts

1. Wachter, MD, Robert M. *WebM&M* interview with Mr. Boothman, March 2012.
2. Eichhorn, MD, John H., Jeffrey B. Cooper, PhD, David J. Cullen, MD, Ward R. Maier, MD, James H. Philip, MD, and Robert G. Seeman, MD, "Standards for Patient Monitoring During Anesthesia at Harvard Medical School" *JAMA.* August 22, 1986.
3. Hornbein, MD, Thomas F. *JAMA* August 22/29 1986. 256(8). "The Setting of Standards of Care" response piece is signed University of Washington, Seattle.
4. Pronovost Checklist was initiated after an adverse medical event at Johns Hopkins Hospital in 2001.
5. Landro, Laura. "The Secret to Fighting Infections: Dr. Peter Pronovost says it isn't that hard. If only hospitals would do it." Interview, *Wall Street Journal.* March 27, 2011.
6. Gawande, MD, Atul. *The Checklist Manifesto.* Metropolitan Books, 2010.

7. Wachter, MD, Robert M., and P. J. Pronovost. "Balancing 'No Blame' with Accountability in Patient Safety." *New England Journal of Medicine*, October 1, 2009.
8. http://www.ntsb.gov/.
9. Denham, C.R., C.B. Sullenberger, D.W. Quaid, and J.J. Nance. "An NTSB for health care: learning from innovation: debate and innovate or capitulate" *Journal Patient Safety*. 8(1):13–14 March 8, 2012.
10. Todd, James S. "Lifting the burden of malpractice: Take it out of the courts." *Chicago Sun Times*: January 17, 1988.

Chapter 5: Behind the AMA Curtain
1. Starr, Paul. *The Social Transformation of American Medicine: The rise of a sovereign profession and the making of a vast industry.* Basic Books: 1982.
2. FSMB. *State of the States: Physician Regulation 2009.* A report of the Federation of State Medical Boards, Dallas, Texas. 2009.
3. O'Shea, Margaret. "Doctors told not to tamper with lawsuit witnesses." *Greenville News*, 1992.
4. New Jersey Law Revision Commission, Medical Peer Review Final Report Memorandum, August 30, 2004.
5. Barzun, Jacques. "The Professions Under Siege." *Harpers*, October 1978.

Chapter 6: What a Collage of Book Reviews Tell Us
1. Makary, MD, Marty. *Unaccountable: What Hospitals Won't Tell You and How Transparency Can Revolutionize Healthcare.* Bloomsbury Press, 2012.
2. Kussin, MD, Steven Z. *Doctor, Your Patient Will See You Now.* Rowman and Littlefield Publishers, Inc., 2012.
3. Sullenberger, Captain Chesley "Sully." *Highest Duty: My Search for What Really Matters.* HarperCollins Publishers, 2009.
4. Gawande, MD, Atul. *The Checklist Manifesto.* Metropolitan Books, 2010.
5. Torinus, Jr., John, *The Company That Solved Health Care.* BenBella Books, Inc., 2010.
6. Topol, MD, Eric, *The Creative Destruction Of Medicine: How the Digital Revolution Will Create Better Health Care.* Basic Books, NY, 2012.
7. Wachter, MD, Robert M. and Kaveh G. Shojania, MD, *Internal Bleeding: The Truth Behind America's Terrifying Epidemic of Medical Mistakes* by Rugged Land LLC, 2004. Second Edition 2012.
8. Herzlinger, Regina, *Who Killed Health Care:* America's $2 Trillion Medical Problem and the Consumer-Driven Cure. McGraw-Hill, 2007.
9. Lundberg, MD, George D. *Severed Trust*: Why American Medicine Hasn't Been Fixed—and What We Can Do About It. Basic Books, 2001.

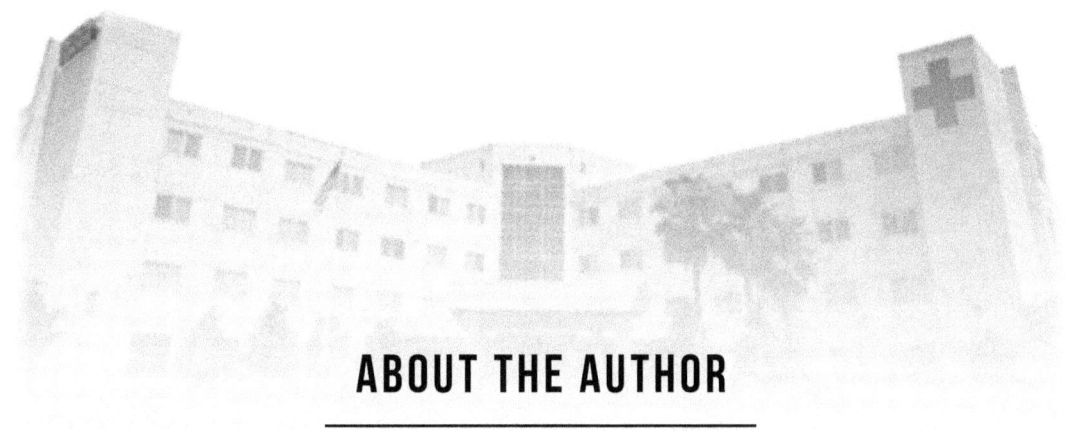

ABOUT THE AUTHOR

Dr. Ira E. Williams has more than fifty years of experience in healthcare as a board certified oral and maxillofacial surgeon and anesthesiologist. He served as president of the Wisconsin Oral Surgery Society, 1977–79, member of a hospital executive committee (1974–76, 1980–82), and experienced in medical peer review and medical malpractice litigation as an expert witness (initially as second surgeon multiple times).

Medical training highlights include Anesthesia training with Dr. Jay Jacoby (father of recovery rooms, ICU, and Code Blue) who organized the first department of anesthesia at Ohio State University in 1947; the performance of thirty-five autopsies during a six-month pathology rotation; and Dr. Williams solely organized (in Madison, Wisconsin, in 1970) the first major surgical mini-residency for the surgical correction of jaw deformities, which drew oral surgeons from five states and initiated the creation of other mini-residencies throughout the country.

Dr. Williams is a retired United States Air Force major and senior navigator/bombardier. His twenty-four years of military service included active duty assignments in Korea, Japan, Florida, South Carolina, Louisiana, and Arkansas.

He served as squadron commander, Wing Headquarters Squadron, 461st Bomb Wing, Blytheville, AFB, AK; Summary Court Martial officer, Air Force Academy Liaison officer, Air Force reservist and both Tennessee and Wisconsin Air National Guard, and he received a Presidential Unit Citation after the Cuban Missile Crisis (1962).

Dr. Williams is a pilot and has flown a gilder, takeoff to landing. He lives in Greenville, South Carolina.

Other Books by Dr. Ira E. Williams
Misdiagnosed! Why Current Health Care Change is Malpractice, 2010.
First, Do No Harm: The Cure for Medical Malpractice, 2004.

Dr. Williams welcomes your feedback.
Contact him directly for speaking engagements. findtheblackbox@gmail.com http://findtheblackbox.org
http://healhc.com

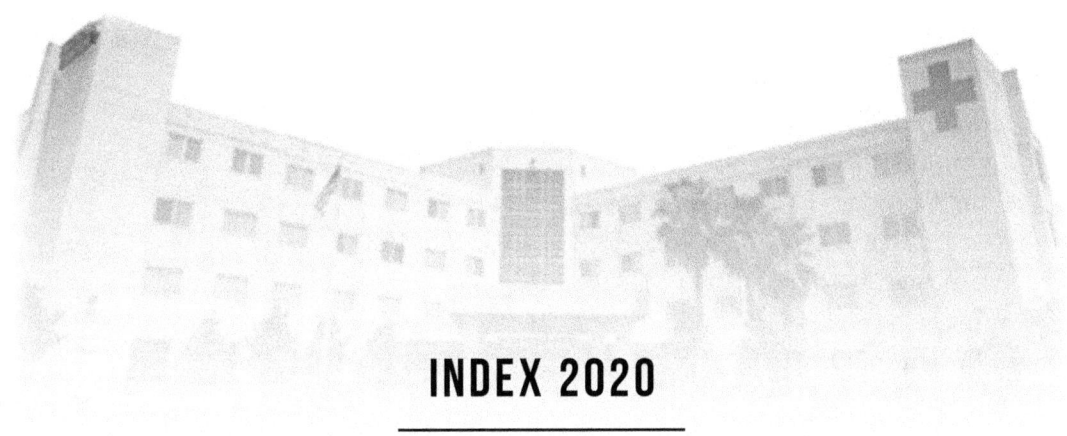

INDEX 2020

Quality of HC Experts
Berwick, Donald, Dr. 1, 2, 31, 46-48, 165, 169
    Institute for Healthcare Improvement (IHI), 43, 47, 52, 165
    Respectful management, 49
    Triple Aim, 52
    Bisognano, Maureen, 48
Boothman, Richard, 56-66, 71, 79, 80, 117, 118, 126, 186
    Anderson, Susan, 60
    Campbell, Skip, 61
    Ypsilanti, 62
Brennan, Troven, Dr. xxxii, xxxiii, 87, 165, 166, 189
    Mello, Michelle, 189
Casssel, Christine, Dr. 47, 163, 164
Charnley, John, Dr 82
Clancy, Carolyn, Dr. 32, 34, 168
    3.1% increase in the quality of care for third year, 32, 168
Corrigan, Janet, xxxi, xxxiii, 2, 36, 41, 47, 163, 168
    Why Have We Not Gotten Further?, 2, 6, 89, 161, 168
    Patient safety is improving only 1% each year, 2
Denham, Charles, 84, 85, 90, 91, 141, 169
    NTSB for HC, 84, 85, 142, 169
    Nance, John, 84, 85, 87, 159, 169
    Quaid, Dennis, xxvii, 84, 85, 87, 141, 159, 169
Fisher, Elliott, 1, 2, 23, 168
Flexner, Abraham, (Report), 12, 55, 172, 173
Gawande, Atul, Dr.1, 2, 48, 75, 80, 83, 88, 136, 145, 161, 169
    Checklist Manifesto, 145
Kizer, Keeneth, Dr. 46, 167
    Never event, 46, 167
Leape, Lucian, Dr. xxxi-xxxiii, 2, 31, 47, 87, 131-133, 143, 163, 165, 168, 189

Makary, Marty, Dr. 14, 20-24, 46, 66, 131, 136, 157, 158, 161, 163, 169
McClellan, Mark, 1, 2, 168
McGlynn, Elizabeth, PhD xxxiv, 7, 168
    Rand Corporation, 7, 168
Pronovost, Peter, Dr. 46, 71, 77, 79, 88, 135, 153, 156, 168
    Balancing "No Blame", 152, 153, 168
    Surgery Journal, 46
Rush, Benjamin, Dr. 115
Semmelweis, Ignaz, Dr. xxxvii, 81, 192, 193
    Lister, Joseph, Dr, xxxvii, 82
Sullenberger, Sully, xxvii-xl, 2, 84, 87, 89, 91, 97, 141-143, 169, 193
    Feith, Greg, 142
Wachter, Robert, Dr xxxvi, xxxviii, 2, 23, 24, 31-34, 36-44, 47, 56, 77-80, 83-86, 136, 152, 157-161, 168-170, 186, 193
    Is Pt. Safety Flickering Out?, 41, 170, 193
    Flansbaum, Brad, 43
    Golden Era of Patient Safety, 41
    Gunderman, Richard 43
    IHI's Global Trigger Tool, 43
    Maslow hierarchy of needs, 43
    Morrison, Ian, 44
    Root Cause Analysis, 41
    Sexton, Bryan, 42

Quality of HC Components
Federal
Department of Health & Human Services (DHHS), 30
    AHRQ, 31, 34, 35, 158, 168
    Web M&M, 34-36, 47, 56, 158
    Evidence Based Medicine, 32-33
    Evidence Based Practice, 32-33
    Sackett, David, Dr. 32
HCQIA – 86, 117
Institute of Medicine (IOM), 28-41, 155, 165, 166, 169
    To Err Is Human, 25-39, 86, 155, 165, 166
    Crossing Quality Chasm, 30-37, 156
National Patient Data Bank, 46

Other
Confirmation bias, xxxiv
DNV Healthcare, 14

Harmonization, xxxiv
Leapfrog Group, 26, 47
MacArthur Foundation, 73, 74, 76
National Quality Forum (NQF), 2, 35-37, 45-49, 71, 166, 168
PECORI, 27, 50-52, 154
Robert Wood Johnson Foundation, 95, 96
Texas Institute for Medical Technology (TMIT), 84, 85, 87
World Health Organization (WHO), 53, 71, 73, 74, 77, 85-88

States
Haley, Nikki, 10, 12, 14, 77, 130, 131, 169, 171-174
Taylor, Spence, Dr. xxxv, 2, 10, 130, 168, 174
    Greenville Hospital System, xxxv, 2, 168
MADD, 3, 6, 128, 190
SC Business Coalition, 49, 152
SC HC Delivery System, 11, 130, 171
    (16 components), 11
SC Hospital Assoc., 13, 74-78, 145, 174
    Thornton Kirby 75
SC Medical Board, 4, 14
SC Law Enforce (SLED), 4
Keck, Tony, 12
Thompson, Governor, 174

Medical Profession
Am. Assoc. Oral & Max Surgeons, 124, 125
    OSMIC Monitor, 124, 125
    Fortress Insurance Company, 124
Am. Bd. Ob/Gyn, 10, 35
    Gluck, Paul, Dr. 35
Am. Col. Legal Medicine, 110
AMA,
    California MICRA-75, 120
    Gold Standard, 120
    JAMA, 66-69, 120, 124, 130, 162
    Litigation Center, 29, 54, 103-111, 130, 143, 166, 167
    LOSER PAYS, 143
    Medical Liability Project, 93, 165
    Medical malpractice tort reform, 118
        (CBO), 119
        Tort Reform NOW!, 120

Will Your Doctor Be There?, 110,167
  Doctor/Oncologist, 126
  Doctor/Son, 126
Bill,
  Congenital hydrocephalus, 100
  NC Court of Appeals, 106
  NC Medical Board, 105-112, 167
  NC Medical Society, 103-112, 167
  Keene, Stephen, 105, 106, 110
  Expert Witness, 105-107
  Neurosurgeon #1, 101-104, 107
  Neurosurgeon #2, 101-107
  Palmisano, Donald, Dr. 89, 110-111, 158, 167
  Res ipsa loquitur, 102
Federation of State Medical Boards, 106-113
  International Association of Medical Regulatory Authorities, 112
Joint Commission, 14, 41, 48, 166
Medical malpractice crisis, 91
Mother's Dying, Someone Do Something! 126
  Doctor/Oncologist, 126
  Doctor/Son, 126
Nat. Patient Safety Foundation, 2, 29, 54, 168
  Hatlie, Martin, 53
Special medical malpractice courts, 91
  Code of Silence, 121
  Common Good, 94
  Barringer, Paul, 95
  Foriet, Jenny, 95
  Gingrich, Newt, 8, 94
    Center for Health Transformation, 96
  Howard, Phillip, 94
  Redding, California 86,
  Wisconsin courts, 92
Sue or Forget It, 47, 65, 127, 130, 142, 143, 177, 178, 186, 192

Medical Centers and Schools
Harvard Anesthesia Department, 66-70, 145, 165
  Cooper, Jeffery, Dr. 66
  Cullen, David, Dr. 66
  Eichhorn, John, Dr. 66
  Maier, Ward, Dr. 66

Philip, James, Dr. 66
Seeman, Robert, Dr. 66
University of Michigan Health System, 56-62, 79, 126
University of Pittsburg Medical Center, 126
University of Washington Medical Center, 127
Virginia Mason Health System – Seattle, 42
    Gary Kaplan, Dr. 42
Arnold School of Public Health, 109
Harvard School of Public Health, xxvii, 20, 25, 69, 74, 112, 165

Books
Can't Is Not An Option, 130
Doctor, Your Patient Will See You Now, 125
    Kussin, Steven, Dr. 135-141
    Captain of the ship, 141
    Hospitalists, 137-140
    Yin and Yang, 139
Highest Duty, 141
Internal Bleeding, 157
    Wachter, Robert, Dr., & Shojania, Kayeh, 157
Medical Malpractice Solutions, 94
Severed Trust, 160
    Lundberg, George, Dr. 160
    Bramstedt, Katrina, 162
    DeAngelis, Catherine, Dr. 162
The Company That Solver Health Care, 146
    Torinus, John, 146
    Mother Teresa, 149
    O'Neill, Paul, 149
    Scandlen, Greg, 149
    Zastrow, Raymond, 152
The Creative Destruction of Medicine, 154-157
    Topol, Eric, Dr. 154
    Health Information Technology (HIT), 155
    Ioannidis, John, 154
    Orszag, Peter, 154
    Schumpeter, Joseph, 154
The Professions Under Siege, 122
    Barzun, Jacques, 122
    Esprit de corps, 123
The Transformation of Medicine, 109

Starr, Paul, 109,187
Unaccountable, 13, 14, 21, 66, 118, 131, 169
    D'Angelo Fellmeth, Julie, 134
    O'Kolo, Patrick, Dr. 135
Who Killed Healthcare?, 8, 146, 159
    Herzlinger, Regina, 8, 146, 159
    Coburn, Tom, Dr. 159

Media Outlets
Chicago Sun Times, 93
Greenville Journal, xxxv
Greenville News, 75, 105
    Doctors told not to tamper, 114
New York Times, 1, 74, 154, 168
Wall Street Journal, xxxviii, 8, 20, 68, 166
    Elliott, J.H., xxxviii
    Hay, William Anthony, xxxviii
    Landro, Laura, 20,71
    Perry, Rick, 8
    Romney, Mitt, 8
Wisconsin State Journal, 68
Harpers Magazine, 124
Health Affairs, 156,169
Parade Magazine, 54
    A Day in the Life of a Country Doctor, 54
    Burton, Marion, Dr. 54
    Keys, Janice, 54
    Koller, Lillian, 54
    McMahan, Howard, 54
    Templeton, Catherine, 54
Time Magazine, 71
Journal of Oral Surgery, 83
Journal of Patient Safety, 84, 85
Journal PLoS Medicine, 154
New England Journal of Medicine, 74, 79, 131, 134, 168
New Jersey Law Revisions Commission, 115, 189
    Scheutzow, Susan, 115
Patient Safety & Quality Healthcare Journal, 53
    Sheridan, Susan, 53
    We're Not Your Enemy, 53
PBS, 110, 167

Suarez, Ray, 110
60 Minutes, 14,160
    Health Management Associates, 14

Quotes
Machiavelli, Nicolo, 7, 15, 55
Rand, Ayn, xl
Santayana, George, 110, 188
Schopenhauer, Arthur, 171

Personal
461st Bomb Wing, 18
Anderson, Rudolph, Major 98, 144
Autopsies, 111, 160
Copenhagen, Denmark, 98, 144
Cuban Crisis, 98, 144
Dunkirk, 82
Hinds, Edward, Dr. 83
IRPR, 178-186
Jacoby, Jay, Dr., 70
Kelly, Stuart, Dr., 15
Kennedy, President, 12, 16, 98, 144
    Sputnik, 12
Kennedy, Rosemary, 16
Korea, 18,76,77,
ON Button, 179
Peer Review Committee, 182
Presidential Unit Citation, 98, 144
Puckett, Kenneth, Airman, 19
Sully, 97, 143
Wolfe, Tom, 80
Yeager, Chuck, General, 80

www.ingramcontent.com/pod-product-compliance
Lightning Source LLC
LaVergne TN
LVHW081455060526
838201LV00051BA/1804